GW00319357

OPTIMUM NUTRITION

Patrick Holford

ION
PRESS

PATRICK HOLFORD started his academic career in the field of psychology. While completing his bachelor's degree in experimental psychology at the University of York he researched the role of nutrition in mental illness. His fascination with this subject led him to the United States, where he studied the work of Dr.Carl Pfeiffer MD PhD at the Brain Bio Center, and other leading figures in nutritional medicine. He has since carried out research into mental health, pre-menstrual syndrome, athletic performance, hair mineral analysis and the importance of trace elements such as zinc. In 1984 he founded the Institute for Optimum Nutrition, a non profit-making independent centre for the research and practice of nutrition, where he now teaches and practices.

He is one of Britain's leading nutritional authors writing for a number of major national publications and frequently appearing on radio and television. His books include The Whole Health Manual, Elemental Health, The Family Nutrition Workbook, The Better Pregnancy Diet, The Metabolic Diet, The Energy Equation, Supernutrition for a Healthy Heart and How To Protect Yourself from Pollution.

First published in 1992
by ION Press, London.

© Patrick Holford 1992

Illustrations and cover: Christopher Quayle
Lay-out: Heather James

All rights reserved. No part of this publication may be reproduced, stored in a retrieval system, or transmitted, in any form or by any means, electronic, mechanical, photocopying, recording or otherwise, without the prior written permission of the publishers.

ISBN 1 87096 05 3

Printed and bound in Great Britain by
RAP Ltd, Rochdale
on recycled paper

CONTENTS

ACKNOWLEDGEMENTS

There is always someone behind the scenes 'without whom this book couldn't have been written'. My special thanks go to Chris for the beautiful cover and illustrations and Heather for her design, layout and indispensable support, Sonya for her speedy typing, Anne, Kate and Brenda-Jean for letting me get on with it, and Janet for her proofing. I also wish to thank Kate Neil, Nicky Giles, Liz Lorente, Anne Pelter, Anne Gains and the Campaign for Health Through Food for permission to use their delicious recipes in Chapter 15, and Ruth Joseph for her help in Chapter 10.

I also wish to acknowledge and thank most sincerely Dr. Stephen Davies, Dr. Jeffrey Bland, Dr. Michael Colgan, Dr. Linus Pauling, Dr. Roger Williams, Dr. Carl Pfeiffer, Professor Michael Crawford, Professor Derek Bryce-Smith, Dr. Neil Ward and many other fine scientists and practitioners whose insight and pioneering work has helped to establish the concept of optimum nutrition and has certainly been an inspiration to me. Finally, a special thanks to my first teachers, Brian and Celia Wright, who introduced me to this exciting field in 1978.

Guide to abbreviated measures

1 gram (g) = 1,000 milligrams (mg) = 1,000,000 micrograms (mcg)
Most vitamins are measured in milligrams or micrograms. Vitamins A, D and E are also measured in International Units (iu), a measurement designed to provide standardisation of the different forms of these vitamins that have different potencies.

1mcg of retinol *or* 2mcg of beta carotene = 3.3iu of vitamin A
1mcg of vitamin D = 40iu
1mg of vitamin E= approx. 1iu of alpha tocopherol

For research purposes, measurements of minerals in the blood are expressed in micrograms per decilitre (mcg/dl); those in the hair in parts per million (ppm).

References

Over 200 references from respected scientific literature have been referred to in this book. A full list of these references, listed in sequential order with the numbers corresponding to the subscript numbers in the text, is available from the Institute for Optimum Nutrition, 5 Jerdan Place, London, SW6 1BE. Please send £2 and an SAE.

This book is dedicated to you -
the promoter of your own health.

INTRODUCTION

In 1977 I met two extraordinary nutritionists, Brian and Celia Wright. They explained to me, over an enormous bowl of salad and some 'soya sausages', followed by a handful of vitamin pills, how most disease was the result of sub-optimum nutrition. I found this hard to swallow, but being an adventurous spirit, asked them to devise me a diet. There I was, a university student studying psychology, eating a wheat-free virtually vegetarian diet, masses of fruit and vegetables, and taking a handful of supplements, which were shipped from America since they were not available in Britain at that time. A far cry from the usual fish and chips and a pint of bitter! My colleagues, my friends and my family thought I was crazy. But I persisted.

Within two months I lost a stone in weight, which has never returned; my skin, which had resembled a lunar landscape, cleared up; my regular migraines virtually vanished; but most noticeable of all was the extra energy. I no longer needed so much sleep, my mind was so much sharper and my body full of vitality. I started to investigate this 'optimum nutrition'. Being a psychology student I looked up research on the greatest problem in mental health today, schizophrenia. There, in the scientific journals, was clear proof that 'optimum nutrition' produced results better than drugs and psychotherapy combined. A pioneer in this field, Dr. Carl Pfeiffer, an American doctor and psychiatrist, was claiming an 80% remission rate! I was fascinated and, before long, went to America to see for myself.

Dr. Carl Pfeiffer, a brilliant man who spent most of his life studying the chemistry of the brain, had a massive heart attack when he was 51. His chances of surviving were very slim, ten years at the absolute most - if he had a pacemaker fitted. He decided not to, and spent his next 30 years pursuing and researching optimum nutrition. "It is my firmly held belief" he told me "that with an adequate intake of micro-nutrients - essential substances we need to nourish us - most chronic diseases would not exist. Good nutritional therapy is the medicine of the future. We have already waited too long for it."

The optimum nutrition approach is not new. Many great visionaries have embraced it. In 390AD Hippocrates said "Let food be your medicine and medicine be your food". Edison, in the 20th century said "The doctor of the future will give no medicine but will interest his patients in the care of the human frame, diet, and the cause and prevention of disease." In 1960 one of the geniuses of our time, twice Nobel prize winner Dr.Linus Pauling,   coined the phrase 'orthomolecular nutrition'. He proposed that, by giving the body the right (ortho) molecules most disease would be eradicated. Optimum nutrition, he believes, is the medicine of tomorrow. Now, thirty two years later and still actively researching at the age of 91, he is stronger than ever in his conviction.

In 1984 I founded the Institute for Optimum Nutrition in London to research and promote optimum nutrition. We extolled the virtues of health eating and vitamin supplements, warned of the dangers of lead in petrol, additives in food, pollutants in water, and of fried food and free radicals, and the value of anti-oxidant vitamins A, C and E, and minerals such as selenium and zinc. It is gratifying that many of these ideas have been taken to heart. Lead in petrol and additives in food are on the way out, tighter controls on pollutants in water are on the way in. Last year the Department of Health released £1.65 million to research the optimal intake of vitamins A, C and E to prevent cancer and heart disease. Optimum nutrition is, it seems, an ideas whose time has come.

The purpose of this book is to show you how to achieve vibrant health and resistance to disease through optimum nutrition. PART ONE explains the principles of optimum nutrition which necessitates a whole new definition of health, healthcare and medicine. PART TWO proves the benefits of optimum nutrition based on the latest breakthroughs in nutritional science. PART THREE shows you how to put optimum nutrition into practice with a step-by-step guide to help you improve your diet and design your own supplement programme.

Fifteen years have passed since I first discovered optimum nutrition. In that time literally thousands of scientific papers have been published proving the potency of optimum nutrition, and virtually none that negate it. I am now completely convinced that the concept of optimum nutrition is the greatest step forward in medicine this century, and, if applied from an early age, is a guarantee for a long and healthy life.

Patrick Holford

PART 1

THE PRINCIPLES OF OPTIMUM NUTRITION

1
WHAT IS HEALTH ?

There exists for all of us the tangible and achievable experience of a profound sense of well-being. This is characterised by a consistent, clear and high level of energy, an emotional balance, a sharp mind, a desire to maintain physical fitness and a direct awareness of what suits our bodies, what enhances our health, and what our needs are in any given moment. This state of health includes a resilience to infectious diseases, a virtual impossibility of contracting many of the major killer diseases such as heart disease and most forms of cancer, and results in a considerable slowing down of the ageing process. At its most profound level health is not merely the absence of pain or tension, but a joy of living, a real appreciation of what it is to have a healthy body with which to taste the many pleasures of this world

For me, this is not a belief but an experience which I both have and have witnessed in so many other people with whom I have worked over the past thirteen years since I started to pursue 'optimum nutrition'. Health has not been a static state, but an endless journey of learning about myself from the diseases and imbalances that I have suffered, and a continuing discovery of even higher and clearer levels of energy.

Out of my own experiences and those gained from working with thousands of people suffering from virtually every category of disease I am totally convinced that, through optimum nutrition, exercise, living in the right environment, and being willing to change obsolete beliefs and behaviours that create tension and stress, virtually all disease can be eliminated without recourse to drugs or surgery, except perhaps when a serious disease state is already well established.

The Four Causes of Disease

If this is so, why do we spend over £2,000 million on drugs per annum? Why, as a nation, are we so sick? In my opinion there are only four basic causes of disease: ignorance, resistance to change, choice and bad luck.

Most of us are ignorant about how to maintain health. This isn't taught in schools, our parents don't teach us, our doctors don't teach us, and advertising and commercial concerns actively promote our ignorance for their own financial gains. Fortunately we can remedy this by reading, by studying and by trying things out. Somewhere along this road we become more and more responsible for our own health and, instead of putting our life in the hands of practitioners, we can use the knowledge of practitioners to help deepen our own experience of health.

Yet, even when we have the knowledge we don't always apply it. Why? Where does resistance to change come from? Or rather, where does the motivation to make the effort to change bad habits come from? It comes from the memory, hope or trust that there is something better than this - that there is a state of well-being that is worth making the effort to reach. Of course, many of us only change our bad habits when they are causing us so much pain that we can't continue a normal life. Life therefore forces us to make changes if we're not ready to make the changes before heavy duty suffering sets in.

Even so, there are times when, consciously or unconsciously, we choose to be ill to fulfill some need. The hyperactive workaholic who gets migraines as a way of shutting down the mind, the adolescent who develops anorexia to avoid growing up, the child who develops a tummy ache in order to miss school - these are common examples.

Finally there's bad luck. We are all born with certain defects. For some these are severe, such as the many genetic diseases. We may, in the course of our life, have a debilitating accident, or suffer a stage of acute illness that causes permanent or long-term damage, and for too many people, there is simply the lack of means to attain health, be it food, water, sanitation and so on. I prefer to think of these things as obstacles rather than bad luck, since it is only through the overcoming of obstacles that we learn. St. Francis's prayer was "Give me the patience to accept the things I cannot change, the strength to change the things I can and the wisdom to know the difference." These qualities are certainly abundant in those whose circumstances have unavoidably resulted in suffering and disease.

The Four Pillars of Health

With adequate knowledge, the means and the will to change it is inevitable that your health will improve as you build up a solid foundation of healthy living. The four pillars of healthy living are:

1 Optimum nutrition, which seeks to perfect the balance of the body on a chemical level;
2 Fitness, which seeks to perfect balance on a physical level;
3 Attitude, which seeks to perfect balance on a mental and emotional level;
4 Environment, which seeks to perfect the environment in which we live.

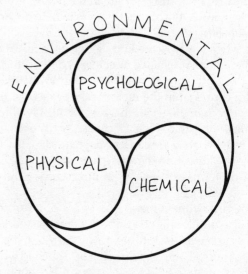

Figure 1 *The Four Pillars of Health*

Body, Mind and Spirit

Although we like to conceive of these realms - chemical, physical, psychological and environmental - as separate, in truth they are inseparable. Yet if you ask a chemist, an anatomist and a psychologist to define where the mind starts and the body ends they will find that the two are interconnected. Every thought is a chemical event which has the capacity of altering the physical tension of the body. Every meal passes through physical organs where it is chemically digested until its constituents can be used to provide the fuel for thought. Yet even though this concept is so obvious it is extraordinary how many physicians deny the importance of psychological factors in disease, and how many psychologists deny the role of nutrition in conditions like schizophrenia and anorexia nervosa.

In the same way we cannot separate ourselves from our environment, as humanity is having to learn fast. Did you know that there are as many micro-organisms inside you as there are body cells? Have you ever stopped to think who you are? Are you your body cells, are you your brain, are you the bacteria in your gut? If someone took away one of your brain cells, or one of your fingers would you feel less 'you'? Whoever we are we live inside this body and express ourselves through it and in that sense our body is our first environment. Our home and workplace represent our next most immediate environment, followed by the world, and then the universe. Again it is impossible to draw the line between us and the environment. Yet so many people still find it hard to believe that pesticides, pollution and electricity pylons could affect our health.

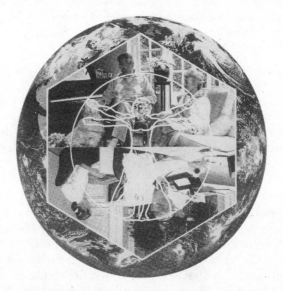

Figure 2 Different Levels of Your Environment

We could add an extra dimension to our model which would encompass 'subtle medicine' including homeopathy, acupuncture and healing. These work on a different or 'subtle' dimension, not in the sense of having a small effect, but in the sense of not influencing health directly through the realms of the chemistry, physics or psychology of a human being. The basis of these approaches includes another dimension. This, of course, is controversial in conventional scientific circles where we would like to be able to explain everything without recourse to concepts that do not fit in with our current models: However, the fact is that the models of homeopathy and acupuncture are being proven scientifically, and such treatments are being proven to have benefit. In due course these 'black sheep' will no doubt stimulate the necessary expansion of our scientific understanding.

Modern Man Is Not Healthier

As limited as our scientific understanding is, it is sad to see how poorly we apply the scientific advances that have been made. We have developed ways of analysing down to a billionth part any component of the human organism. We have developed extraordinary diagnostic skills and methods of investigation, yet, despite this, we are not much healthier. For all our technology, a man ages 45 today can expect to live for two more years than the same man in 1920; until 74, instead of 72. Why is this?

Ego Medicine

I believe that much of today's medicine, much of our pursuit of health, is misdirected. Instead of educating people about diet, fitness, attitude and the environment, which should be the job of health practitioners, most of today's medicine operates a 'patch up' service using powerful drugs and surgical procedures which themselves harm the body, without adequate explanation of the cause of the imbalance or the way in which the treatment works and the potential side effects. It is as if some practitioners believe themselves to be in control of other people's health with their high-tech equipment and panorama of flashy medicines. Gone is any sense of wonder or humility towards this extraordinary organism, the human body, which has been shaped over millennia and continues to amaze us through the complexity of its design. Likewise, some patients believe that health and even life itself can be bought, if you've got enough money. They demand the best medical care, life extension programmes, face lifts, muscle building regimes, and, just in case these don't work, a good insurance policy. Often there is a laziness in this arrogance - a willingness to give the responsibility for one's health to a practitioner rather than accept the responsibility oneself. There is also a laziness of thought, which is a major obstacle to the advancement of science and knowledge, in that one accepts a system without testing and challenging it with an open mind.

Zen and the Art of Body Maintenance

Narrow vision exists as much within complementary medicine as it does within conventional medicine. I am reminded of the book, Zen and the Art of Motorcycle Maintenance, which in essence proposed that there were two predominant personality types: the romantics - arty, ethereal, feeling people; and the technocrats - scientific, futuristic, thinking people. The romantics love 'yin-yang' balanced diets, healing workshops and crystals and the technocrats love biochemical tests, complicated vitamin programmes, computers and graphs. The romantics believe that all the world's problems would be solved if enough of us held hands and visualised white light flowing to all humanity. The technocrats believe that we will solve the world's problems through a careful analysis of the situation and by making technological advances. Both of these views contain some truth, but both can equally blind us to an expanded view and experience of health. I believe that any approach to health or nutrition should:

1 Fundamentally make sense at a gut level;
2 Be proved through one's own experience
   and when applied to others;
3 Be capable of proof using proper scientific method;
4 Be in harmony with the environment.

These truths are nothing new, but they are often forgotten. They have been expressed throughout history, from the time of Hippocrates right up to the twentieth century. They are succinctly expressed by the constitution of the World Health Organisation which states that "Health is a state of complete physical, mental and social well-being and not merely the absence of disease or infirmity. The enjoyment of the highest attainable standard of health is one of the fundamental rights of every human being without regard to race, religion, political belief and economic or social condition." If that is the goal, what is the means?

2
WHAT IS OPTIMUM NUTRITION?

Optimum nutrition is very simply giving yourself the best possible intake of nutrients to allow your body to be as healthy and to work as well as it possibly can. It is not a set of rules. For example, you don't have to be vegetarian or take supplements or not eat any particular food, although for some people such advice would be appropriate. Your needs are completely unique and depend on a whole host of factors from the strengths and weaknesses you were born with right up to the effects your current environment has on you. You only have to look at the tremendous variation in the way we look, our talents and personalities to realise that our nutritional needs are not likely to be identical. No one diet works for us all.

Biochemical Individuality
At the same time there are many principles that apply to us all. We may be different, but we're not that different. We all need vitamins for example, but the amount we need for peak performance varies from individual to individual. This principle of biochemical individuality is the first principle of the optimum nutrition approach. Biochemical Individuality was first succinctly proposed by Dr.Roger Williams in 1956.[1] Dr. Williams was one of the grandfathers of optimum nutrition and true to form was actively teaching, writing and researching well into his nineties. In his book, Biochemical Individuality, he showed how our organs are different shapes and sizes, how we have different levels of enzymes, (the chemicals that

break other chemicals down, for example digesting food) and different needs for protein, vitamins and minerals. Ten-fold differences in the requirement for vitamins from person to person is not at all uncommon. For example, a comparison of the level of vitamin A in the blood of 92 individuals found a 30-fold difference.[2] This result suggests a wide range among people in their need for vitamin A. Some of us, therefore are good at digesting protein, but not fat, or need more of a particular vitamin than the average diet can supply.

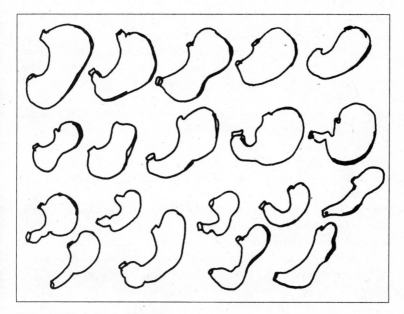

Figure 3 *Variation in Stomachs*

Nutrition is a Function of the Environment

You may then ask why are we different or, conversely, why are we similar? The answer to these questions defines the second principle of optimum nutrition. We are shaped by our environment, which includes the nutrition we receive from our environment.

In the short span of your life, how you were nourished as a child affects your needs later in life. For example, pregnant rats deprived of zinc for a short period during pregnancy give birth to babies with a weakened immune system, which stays weak for life despite adequate zinc nourishment. Their offsprings in turn have a weakened

17

immune system and an extra requirement for zinc.[3] The same seems to be true for baby humans too. Likewise, if you eat a lot of wheat as a child you may be more likely to become wheat allergic later in life. In America, where corn is the predominant grain, it is the number one food allergy. In Britain, wheat, our staple food, is top of the list. Americans get hayfever from ragweed pollen, a common weed, while in Britain we are more likely to react to pollen from grasses. Is it any wonder that, in the twentieth century, when the average person breathes in two grams of solid pollution, eats 12lbs of chemical food additives, and has up to a gallon of pesticides sprayed on the fruit and vegetables they consume each year, that simply eating a 'well balanced' diet is not enough?

The long-term effects of our environment are much more significant. The human race has evolved over millions of years. That perspective is so easy to forget when we become wrapped up in our day to day problems. When the earth quakes, volcanoes erupt and famines strike we get a sense of how impotent we are compared to the unstoppable forces of nature. These forces designed and shaped us. Being tree dwelling apes in ancestry infants keep to this day the gripping reflex for hanging on to branches. Like all tree dwelling animals young humans are so difficult to house train compared to den dwelling creatures like dogs who would never soil their den for fear of attracting predators. When stressed, our blood actually coagulates. Why? Because stress prepares us to fight or take flight and fighting often involves wounds that heal more quickly if blood is thicker. These were the stresses of our ancestors, not mortgages, traffic jams and marital rows. Yet our blood still thickens.

Evolutionary Dynamics

This is the third principle of optimum nutrition - the understanding that we have evolved over millions of years, in line with our environment, and that all we need to do is understand what our natural design is and conform to it. Dr. Michael Colgan, one of America's top nutritional scientists, calls this principle evolutionary dynamics.[4] This principle has been incorporated into a whole new understanding of the origins of man, expounded in the book The Driving Force, by Professor Michael Crawford and David Marsh.[5] It is no surprise to find that these scientists themselves pursue optimum nutrition.

Looked at from this perspective it becomes obvious that many of the things we do are against our natural design. For example, we go to sleep because levels of adrenalin, a stimulating chemical, start to drop, and serotonin levels in the brain, a relaxant, start to rise. In the morning, light enters through translucent portions of the skull and stimulates the release of adrenalin. In this way we wake up refreshed and alert. Not so if you sleep with your curtains excluding all light, and wake to the sound of the alarm clock. How many coffees (adrenal stimulants) do you need to get going then? We have not been designed to smoke, to consume alcohol, to eat refined sugar and fibreless diets, cooked and processed foods, to breathe polluted air, to drink polluted water or to live in a constant state of stress. Is it any wonder that we are short changed on health?

Sub-Optimum Nutrition is the Rule in Nature

But don't get the idea that our ancestors were optimally nourished. All species compete for nutrients. Those that do well flourish, those that do badly become extinct. There is a necessary balance. For example, yeasts, present even in the air around us and on many foods, are not optimally nourished otherwise the stuff would be all over the place! There has also been a tendency in nature for dominant species to multiply, consuming all the nutrients in the environment, and then to die off from starvation, or to adapt to consume other resources. Since other factors in the environment are changing, for example, the weather, there is a natural variation or individuality in most species that protects them from sudden extinction due to environmental changes. Some people, for example, are better adapted to hot or cold climates. Perhaps the dinosaurs became extinct because they couldn't adapt to rapid climactic changes, like those predicted to occur in our lifetime.

These historical truths are so important for our understanding of optimum nutrition and for our future survival. Mankind now has the ability to manipulate the environment. We can choose what we eat. We even know, in broad terms, what will make us healthy. We also know, in broad terms, how to live and how to grow food while maintaining a balance with the animal and vegetable kingdom and the world in which we live. In other words, we have the ability to alter the evolution of ourselves and our species - humanity.

Will we choose to nourish ourselves in a way that does not plunder the resources of the earth and our co-habitants? Or will we continue to pollute, overpopulate and plunder the earth? If we choose the latter the earth and those species best adapted to the changes will continue, but humanity may not. If we choose the former, what a wonderful world this could be. Good planets are, after all, hard to find.

So what is optimum nutrition? It is very simply giving yourself the best possible intake of nutrients to allow your body to be as healthy and to work as well as it possibly can, in other words to conform to its natural design. It is based on an understanding of the following principles:

1 Biochemical individuality - your needs are unique.
2 Nutrition and the environment are interconnected.
3 Evolutionary dynamics -we have been shaped over millennia.

This means much more than simply eating a so-called 'well balanced diet', as the next chapter explains. The results are also much more than the avoidance of illness, as the rest of this book and your experience as you apply the principles of optimum nutrition will show you.

3

THE MYTH OF THE BALANCED DIET

T he greatest lie in health care today is that "as long as you eat a well balanced diet you get all the nutrients you need". This is a lie because no single piece of research in the last decade has managed to show that people who consider themselves to be eating a well-balanced diet are receiving all the Recommended Daily Amounts (RDA) of vitamins and minerals, let alone those levels of nutrients that are consistent with optimum nutrition. When conventional nutritionists are asked what a well-balanced diet is, they define it as a diet that provides all the nutrients you need. Catch 22. According to Dr. Stephen Davies these people are "nutritional flat-earthers" because they "employ a thought process akin to that which was adopted by the original 'flat-earthers', those who maintained that the world was flat, rather than round, despite overwhelming evidence to the contrary."[1] The reality is that the vast majority of us are deficient in a number of essential nutrients, which includes vitamins, minerals, essential fatty acids, and amino acids, the constituents of protein. Deficient, means 'not efficient', in other words that you are not functioning as efficiently as you could because you have an inadequate intake of one or more nutrients. If this comes as a shock consider the following facts.

1 RDA's are not optimum. According to the National Academy of Sciences, who set US RDA's "RDA's are neither minimal requirements nor necessarily optimal levels of intake".[2] In the UK, government funds research to define the optimum intake of vitamins C and E to

protect against cancer and heart disease, in recognition of the fact that RDA levels are not necessarily optimum,[3] Factors considered to raise one's requirements considerably above RDA levels include alcohol consumption,[4] smoking,[5] exercise habits, pregnancy, times of stress including puberty and premenstrual phases, pollution, and special dietary habits, for example vegetarianism.

2 RDA's vary from country to country. A five-fold variation from one country to another is not at all uncommon. For example, in Holland the RDA for vitamin A is 333 units, while in Switzerland it's 5,500 units. Why the difference?

3 RDA's don't exist for many essential nutrients. There are 45 known essential nutrients. In Britain RDA's exist for only seven of these.

4 The majority of people do not achieve RDA levels from their diet. A government survey in 1990 showed that the average person does not get the RDA for iron.[6] An independent survey in 1985 found over 90 per cent of people consumed less than the US RDA for vitamin B6 and folic acid.[7] A government report stated that 10 per cent of the British population consume less than the 30mg of vitamin C, the UK RDA, while in many other countries the RDA is set at 75mg.[8]

5 Food does not contain what you think it contains. Most of these surveys are based on recording what people eat and looking up what those foods contain in standard text books. But do they take into account that an orange can contain anything from 180mg of vitamin C to nothing?[9] A 100g serving of spinach can contain from 158mg of iron to 0.1mg depending on where it's grown. Wheatgerm can contain from 21ius of vitamin E to 3.2ius. Carrots, that reliable source of vitamin A, can provide a massive 18,500ius down to a mere

Variations in nutrient content in common foods (per 100g of food)		
Vitamin A	in carrots	70 to 18,500iu
Vitamin B5	in wholewheat flour	0.3 to 3.3mg
Vitamin C	in oranges	0 to 116mg
Vitamin E	in wheatgerm	3.2 to 21iu
Iron	in spinach	0.1 to 158mg
Manganese	in lettuce	0.1 to 16.9mg

Figure 4

70ius. Store an orange for two weeks and its vitamin C content will be halved. Boil a vegetable for 20 minutes and 50 per cent of its B vitamins will be gone.[10] Refine brown flour to make white and 78 per cent of the zinc, chromium and manganese are lost.[11] Today's food is not a reliable source of vitamins and minerals.

6 There is a sliding scale of deficiency. Even if we all ate the RDA levels some people would still show signs of deficiency. For the vast majority these would not be the severe symptoms of scurvy, beriberi or pellagra, but they may well show symptoms such as skin problems, lethargy, poor concentration or frequent infections.

The sad truth is that more suffering is caused by malnutrition, both in the West, and in less developed countries, than by any other cause. According to the US Surgeon General, of the 2.1 million Americans who die each year, 1.5 million, 68 per cent, die from diet related diseases. In Britain 64 per cent of people die from heart disease, strokes and cancer, all of which are clearly associated with dietary excesses, deficiencies or environmental factors. At the Institute for Optimum Nutrition, where I practise, we see people with a wide range of problems including digestive disorders, skin problems, cardiovascular disease, cancer, infections, headaches, hormonal problems, diabetes and so on. We have an improvement rate of 86 per cent according to our clients' assessment, not ours.[12]

So why is it that some nutritionists, doctors, scientists, politicians and food companies wish to lull us into a false sense of security by telling us that all we need to do is eat a 'well-balanced diet'? Why are we told that we don't need supplements, when in truth the majority of people do? Why are so many health professionals willing to deprive their patients of the potent and relatively safe approach of optimum nutrition?

Medical Schools Don't Teach Nutrition

I believe there are three reasons - ignorance, money and resistance to change. A doctor qualifying today is unlikely to have had as much as ten hours tuition in nutrition. Unless a doctor has pursued the study of nutrition out of choice he or she is unlikely to be sufficiently informed to advise about optimum nutrition. It is safer to give no advice or refer to someone who is informed, yet too many doctors advise people not to follow special diets or take supplements. This is especially dangerous during pregnancy since it is now well established that people who are vitamin or mineral deficient are more likely to have underweight babies or babies born with birth abnormalities.[13] Fortunately the British Society of Nutritional Medicine publishes a Journal and hold regular conferences to help doctors become informed about nutrition. Their address is given on page xx.

Nutritional Flat-Earthers

Then there are the flat-earthers who simply won't adjust to the wealth of new knowledge in this field. They argue that if you haven't got scurvy you've got enough vitamin C. If you eat a well-balanced diet you're not deficient. If a test result is normal you're healthy (even though you know you're not). They ignore the effects of pollution, drugs, disease and lifestyle on nutritional needs. Such fixed ideas are "adopted when a paradigm shift is occurring and the emergence of a new paradigm is 'generally preceded by a period of pronounced professional insecurity.' We are currently seeing a paradigm shift in the use of nutrition in the treatment and prevention of disease and sub-optimum function." says Dr. Stephen Davies, chairman of the British Society of Nutritional Medicine. [14]

The Politics of Nutrition

One big reason for hanging on to such out-dated beliefs is money. Before the law was passed enforcing the listing of additives on food packaging we were told they were quite safe. The cost to the food industry to make food without using these cheap chemicals was considerable. Although I hope few people really believe it, the sugar industry continue to tell us that sugar is good for you! The food industry makes money out of using cheap ingredients that don't go off and hopefully are addictive, such as sugar, chocolate and coffee. Did you know that not even a weevil can live off white flour? Can you imagine the financial implications for the food industry if suddenly foods were not allowed to be processed in such a way as to destroy nutrients? Or if the RDAs were doubled, showing just how deficient most foods are? Or if chemical and pesticide residues in food had to be declared? Vested interests do not support the public becoming informed about nutrition if it means you'll buy less of their product. Such vested interests influence us through advertising, the media and political lobbies. It is therefore important to know who the financial sponsors of any organisation are. If they are supported by companies who make money out of less nutritious foods their advice needs to be taken with caution. This applies to the British Nutrition Foundation which advises the government about nutritional policy, yet is itself funded by the major companies producing confectionery, high fat foods, processed meats, food chemicals and alcohol.[15] Within government itself many key MPs are also directors or consultants to major food and chemical companies.[16] The Ministry of Agriculture, Food and Fisheries (MAFF), on the one hand, represent the food industry, and on the other, are responsible for many food issues that affect our health. In an ideal society we would insist on a separate ministry concerned with food and health issues which would not be subject to such conflicts of interest.

So who can you trust? The answer is your own body. If something makes sense, is supported by clear evidence and is safe then try it out and see how you feel. The proof, in nutrition, is in the eating. The next chapter introduces you to your body, from the inside out, and gives you simple ways of knowing what suits you.

4
THE WONDERFUL WORLD WITHIN

N othing created by man compares to the magnificent design of the human body. As you read this book 2.5 million red blood cells are made every second within your bone marrow, in order to keep your body cells supplied with oxygen. Meanwhile your digestive system in producing its daily 10 litres of digestive juices to break down the food you eat, roughly 100 tons in a lifetime, taken through your 'inside skin' the gastrointestinal wall which effectively replaces itself every four days. The health of your gastrointestinal tract is maintained by a team of about 300 different strains of bacteria and other micro-organisms as unique to you as your fingerprint, which exceed the total number of cells in your entire body. Meanwhile, your immune system replaces its entire army every week, and when under viral attack, has the capacity to produce 200,00 new immune cells every minute. Even your outside skin is effectively replaced every month, while most of your body is renewed over a seven year period. Your brain, a mere three pounds of mainly fat and water, is processing information of immense complexity through its trillion nerve cells, each connected to 100,000 others in a network whose connections are formed as our life, and the meaning we attach to it, unfolds.

The energy produced from a small amount of food powers all this unseen activity with plenty spare to heat us and allow a wide range of physical activity. Yet, unlike petrol or nuclear fuel there's no pollution. The only by-products are water and carbon dioxide; each essential for plants which in turn produce carbohydrate, our fuel, and oxygen, the spark that lights our cellular fires. It is estimated that we use only a quarter of a percent of our brain's capacity and, in many cases, half the potential lifespan of our bodies. The design, the capacity and the resilience of the human body is truly awesome.

Yet, unlike a new car, we arrive without a maintenance manual and rely on instructions developed by those who have made their livelihood from a study of the human body. These instructions are in their infancy, a fact which is obvious when you consider how much of medicine is based on giving drugs which poison the body, radiation which burns it and surgery which removes defective parts. Most of us only begin to think about body maintenance when something goes wrong. Yet, due to the body's incredible resilience, most serious diseases like cancer and cardiovascular disease take twenty to thirty years to develop. By the time we notice symptoms it may be too late.

Learning from Experience

When you realise that you are a collection of highly organised cells, designed by the forces of nature, adapting to the changing environment over millions of years, it becomes natural to give your body what it needs with the tangible benefit of health. Experience is, of course, the greatest motivator. If something you eat makes you feel good you're likely to continue eating it, while if something makes you feel bad, you're likely to stop - unless you've become addicted. But there is a problem, or rather a dynamic known as the general adaptation syndrome, that needs first to be understood in order to learn from experience. First described in 1956 by Professor Hans Selye, the general adaptation syndrome proposed three stages of reaction to any event.[1] This can be applied to a cigarette, a food, a stress or a physical activity.

STAGE 1 - THE INITIAL RESPONSE The initial response to any event or substance is the best indicator of whether or not it suits you. Remember your first cigarette, your first alcoholic drink or your first coffee? You're unlikely to remember your first intake of sugar, meat or milk or other foods introduced to you when you were very young.

STAGE 2 - ADAPTATION Very quickly your body learns to adapt. Gone is the pounding heart after a coffee, or coughing after a cigarette. An example of this stage is illustrated by the rise in blood pressure when country dwellers, not exposed to air pollution, move

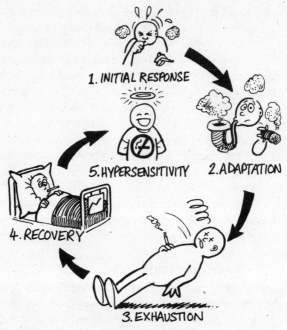

Figure 5 *General Adaptation Syndrome (adapted)*

to a city. There is an immediate increase in blood pressure which later corrects itself. But what is going on behind the scenes? The body is trying to protect itself and, in so doing is in an unseen state of stress. The cells in the lungs of a smoker change form to protect themselves from smoke. Plaque develops in the arteries to repair damaged tissue.

STAGE 3 - EXHAUSTION Continue the insult for long enough and suddenly you're sick. Your energy is gone, your digestion doesn't work, your blood pressure is raised, you develop chest infections or even cancer. The body can't cope, it can't adapt anymore. This is the stage at which most people seek help from a health practitioner.

We could add two further stages to this process.

STAGE 4 - RECOVERY In order for the body to recover it is almost always necessary to avoid or greatly restrict the initial insult and other undesirable substances. This means being as puritanical as possible for a period of time during which you may have to wean yourself off all sorts of things to which you have become addicted or allergic. Generally these are the substances to which you would say "I can give up anything but not my ......". This is the nature of addiction. To help the body recover much larger amounts of vitamins and minerals are needed than would normally be required just to maintain good health.

STAGE 5 - HYPERSENSITIVITY Once recovery has taken place and your body is basically healthy, which can take years, we are effectively back to stage one. But this time, because your diet and lifestyle is much improved you may seem to be hypersensitive and notice reactions to all sorts of things you never reacted to before. Certain wines which contain additives, ordinary foods like wheat or milk, fumes and so on. This is healthy because, like an initial reaction, your body is telling you what suits you. The more you follow this guidance the healthier you will become. In due course, as your reserve strength builds up you can tolerate the odd insult without such hypersensitivity, but by then you will hopefully have learnt (or suffered) enough not to indulge those old bad habits.

Once you understand this cycle and why it is that you can apparently abuse the body without noticeable ill effect, and at other times react strongly to small insults it is easier to interpret what happens to you with clear vision and alter your diet or lifestyle accordingly. Think about the substances that you have suspected may not suit you. What do they have in common? Perhaps there are subtle signs you have chosen to ignore. Here is a list of the most common suspects that many of my clients have found they react to:

Wheat and other grains
Milk and dairy produce
Chocolate
Sugar
Coffee including de-caf
Tea
Alcohol
Yeast based alcohols (beers and wines, not champagne)
Additives in alcohol
Food additives
Cigarettes
Fumes, exhaust, gas fires
Grass pollens

It is interesting that our ancestors, who until relatively recently, were not cultivating grains, nor milking wild animals, were not exposed to any of these.

The Delayed Effect

Another phenomenon worthy of note for those pursuing the 'experiential school of health' is the delayed effect. The General Adaptation Syndrome describes a long-term delayed effect, but for many foods there is a short-term delayed reaction of up to 24 hours before you notice their effect on you. For example, if you eat something very sweet you may feel fine as your blood sugar level rises. But when it plummets four hours later you may fall asleep. Alcohol, for example, has its worst effect many hours later. This is largely because the body, as it tries to detoxify alcohol, actually creates a by-product which induces headaches and nausea. Most substances that are not good for you show an initial reaction within 24 hours of consumption.

A Hairy Bag of Salty Soup

Scientists believe that we, like all other mammals, evolved from the sea. We carry our sea around inside us, which has much the same constituents as the oceans from which we developed. We are 66 per cent water, 25 per cent protein, 8 per cent fat, the rest being carbohydrate plus minerals and vitamins. Saddam Hussein, John Major, Madonna, you and I are all just 66 per cent water. 'Hairy bags of salty soup' said Dr. Michael Colgan, a British born scientist who has pioneered the optimum nutrition approach. Yet if you were to throw all these compounds together you wouldn't end up with a human being. So what is it that makes life happen?

Enzymes - The Keys of Life

Enzymes are the keys to life. Enzymes, although themselves only a collection of the same stuff we're made of, are chemical compounds that turn one substance into another. When you eat an egg enzymes break down the protein into amino acids. These amino acids are small enough to be absorbed into the body where enzymes put them back together again to make body protein. Enzymes turn the food we eat into fuel for every single cell, be it a muscle cell, a brain cell, an immune cell or a blood cell. Enzymes within these cells turn the fuel into usable energy which makes our heart beat, our nerves fire and all other bodily functions take place. Everything in this universe is part of a vast on-going chemical reaction, a dance. Our part, as temporary living organisms, is to provide ourselves and others with the best possible components to allow this process to continue in such a way that we all have a good, enjoyable and long life. That's the way I look at it!

So then the question is "what makes our life giving enzymes function at their peak?" The answer is vitamins and minerals. Nearly all enzymes in the body, of which there are thousands, depend directly or indirectly on the presence of vitamins and minerals. You can't break down or make use of protein, for example, without zinc and vitamin B6. You can't make energy without vitamins B1, B2 and B3 (niacin).

Nutrients Interact

When you understand that the body, and health itself, depend on this vast network of chemical reactions that involve enzymes that are dependent on vitamins and minerals it becomes clear that vitamins and minerals work together. In order for muscle movement to occur we need sufficient fuel (carbohydrate and oxygen) plus vitamin B1, B2, B3, B5, C, iron, calcium and magnesium. There's not much point taking in extra of just one vitamin. That would be like replacing only one dirty spark plug and expecting your car to run smoothly. Yet most medical research into nutrition has done just that, by taking one nutrient and measuring its effect on one aspect of health. As you will see, the research that has produced the most astonishing results in improving energy, mental performance, longevity, fertility and resistance to disease has involved a multi-nutrient approach, recognising that nutrients interact. The next part of this book explains the kind of results that can be achieved and the kind of conditions that can be helped by applying this approach of optimum nutrition.

PART 2

THE BENEFITS OF
OPTIMUM NUTRITION

5

IMPROVING INTELLIGENCE AND MEMORY

When researcher Dr Ruth Harrell heard of a case in which the IQ of a Down's syndrome child went from 20 to 90 points, she decided to explore the ideas that many mentally retarded children might have been born with increased needs for certain vitamins and minerals. In her first study she took 22 mentally retarded children and divided them into two groups. One received vitamin and mineral supplements, the other received placebos (dummy tablets). After four months, the IQ in the group taking the supplements had increased between 5 and 9.6 points; those on placebos showed no change. For the next four months, both groups of children were given the supplements and the average improvement had risen to 10.2 points. Six of the Down's children had improvements of between 10 and 25 IQ points! [1]

The results seemed too good to be true. After all, Down's syndrome is a genetic disease, so how could vitamin supplements increase the intelligence of six of the children so dramatically? This sort of improvement in intelligence would put most of our educationally sub-normal children back in normal classes!

These findings have since been confirmed by three researchers - and contradicted by three more.[2] Why the apparent confusion? Researcher Dr Alex Schauss may have found the answer: it appears that only those children taking thyroid treatment and supplements improved. Neither supplements nor thyroid treatment on their own are expected to help improve intelligence in Down's syndrome patients.

Earlier work in nutrition, such as a study by Kubula in 1960,[3] had shown that increased vitamin status was associated with increased intelligence. He divided 351 students into high and low vitamin C groups, depending on the levels in their blood. The students' IQ was then measured and found to average 113 and 109 respectively: those with higher levels of vitamin C in their blood had an average of 4.5 IQ points more.

The less refined foods you eat the cleverer you are, concluded some researchers at the Massachusetts Institute for Technology. They found that the higher the proportion of refined carbohydrates - such as sugar, commercial cereals, white bread and sweets - in the diet, the lower the IQ score. The difference was almost 25 points![4]

Great improvement in intelligence has also been shown with autistic children,[5] and those with learning difficulties. In a study by Dr Colgan on 16 children with learning and behavioural difficulties, each child had his or her individual nutrient needs determined. Half the children were then given supplements, while the others acted as a control. Each child attended a remedial reading course designed to improve reading age by one year. Over the next 22 weeks teachers carefully monitored the reading age, IQ and behaviour of the children.

Those not taking supplements showed an average increase in IQ of 8.4 points and in reading age of 1.1 years. However, the group on supplements had an improvement in IQ of 17.9 points and their reading age went up by 1.8 years. The most likely explanation, Dr Colgan concluded, was the decline in toxic levels of metals like lead, which are known to have detrimental effects on intelligence.[6]

A number of other studies have proved the connection between lead levels and intelligence. One researcher, Dr Needleman,[7] who has tested thousands of children, has not yet found a single child with high lead who has an IQ above 125. Normally 5 per cent of the population fall above this measurement. An estimated 50 per cent of children in Britain in the 1980's had lead levels high enough to actually impair intelligence. Since the advent of lead-free petrol blood lead levels are fortunately dropping.

Intelligence and Schoolchildren

To test the overall effects of vitamins and minerals on mental performance, Gwillym Roberts, a schoolteacher and nutritionist from ION, and David Benton, a psychologist from Swansea University College, put 60 schoolchildren onto a special multivitamin and mineral supplement designed to ensure an optimal intake of key nutrients.[8] Without their knowledge half these children were placed on a placebo. On analysing the diets of these schoolchildren a significant minority were getting less than the RDA level of at least one nutrient. After eight months on the supplements the non-verbal IQs in those taking the supplements had risen by over 10 points! No changes were seen in those on the placebos, or a control group of students who had not taken any supplements or placebos.

Professor Schoenthaller,[9] from the US, proposed that perhaps a small percentage of schoolchildren were having substantial IQ increases and that, provided the sample size was large enough, the mean IQ difference would be significant.

Clearly, supplements had an effect but the questions raised were: who benefits and why; which nutrients are important at which levels; and how long does it take to get an effect? To answer some of these questions 615 schoolchildren in California were assigned to either a placebo group or one of three 'supplement' groups given approximately 50%, 100% and 200% of the US RDAs for vitamins and minerals. After one month only the 200% RDA group had significantly higher IQ scores than the placebo group. After three months, all supplement groups had higher IQ scores than the placebo group, with the 100% RDA having the highest, and statistically significant, increase. Of this group 45% had an increase in IQ of 15 or more points, compared to the average increase of 4.4 points.

Currently one in five children have learning difficulties, a figure which continues to rise. If this average increase in IQ can be applied to the population at large it would halve the number of children requiring special education.

The message is clear. Keep your vitamin and mineral intake optimum and minimise exposure to pollution if you want to stay smart. Figure 6 summarises the results of some of the studies that have confirmed the link between intelligence and optimum nutrition.

Smart Nutrients

In the last decade a number of individual nutrients have been shown to enhance memory or mental function.[10] However there is little point taking mind-enhancing nutrients if your diet and nutrient intake is not already optimal. This means two things.

Firstly, it means eating a diet low in sugar or adrenal stimulants such as tea or coffee, or fried foods which lead to free radical damage,

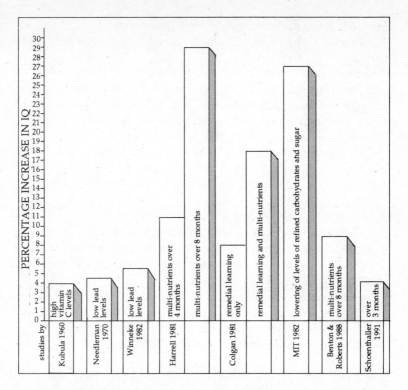

Figure 6   *Effects of Optimum Nutrition on Intelligence*

or aluminium which adversely affects memory. Coffee, alcohol, cigarettes and cannabis have all been shown to impair mental functioning and worsen memory.

Secondly, it means eating a diet (and taking supplements) high in the many nutrients that affect brain function, particularly vitamin B3, B5 (pantothenic acid), B6, B12, choline, calcium, magnesium, zinc, manganese, and chromium and anti-oxidant nutrients A, C, E and selenium. Of these, choline and pantothenic acid in combination are the most important. Vitamin B3 in the form of niacin has been shown to increase memory at doses of 141mg per day.[11] This daily dose, although not dangerous, produces a blushing effect which some people do not like. VitaminB6 and zinc are essential for the formation of many brain neurotransmitters, while calcium and magnesium are involved in nerve transmission. Anti-oxidant nutrients A, C, E and selenium help supply the brain with oxygen and minimise damage from free radicals.

Here are some of the nutrients with 'smart' effects:

Choline is a nutrient found in food, including fish, required for the formation of acetylcholine. It is perhaps the most important neurotransmitter substance in the brain and is intimately associated with memory and intelligence.[12] Choline comes in several forms including choline bitartrate, choline chloride and phosphatidyl choline. Phosphatidyl choline is contained in lecithin.

Pantothenic acid (vitamin B5) is needed to turn choline into acetylcholine in the brain. Pantothenic acid also helps to make stress hormones, reputedly improving one's ability to deal with stressful situations. It is considered non-toxic even in doses of several grams (a gram is 1,000mgs).

Niacin (vitamin B3) is a specific form of vitamin B3 which has a blushing effect in doses above 50mg. At levels of 141mg or more it appears to enhance mental function. Niacin can be toxic at levels well in excess of 1,000mg. Sustained release niacin is best avoided as this has a lower level of toxicity.

Pyroglutamate is an amino acid naturally occurring in vegetables, fruits, dairy and meat. It is very abundant in the cerebro-spinal fluid. It appears to improve mental performance by improving the function of acetylcholine, a neurotransmitter in the brain.[13] No toxicity has yet been reported.

L-glutamine is an amino acid that both helps control neurotransmitters and acts as a fuel for the brain. There is some evidence that it enhances brain function in high doses (3 to 10grams per day) and may reduce craving for alcohol.[14]

DMAE is a naturally occurring nutrient in fish, particularly sardines and anchovies. It is present in the brain in small amounts. It is, in effect, a form of choline which crosses more easily from the blood to the brain and helps produce acetylcholine.It appears to enhance memory, elevate mood and slow down the ageing process.[15] DMAE has a calming and mildly stimulating effect and has been used instead of tranquillizing drugs such as Valium.[16] It is considered non-toxic with the one caution that it should not be given to people who are manic-depressive as it may deepen the depressive phase.

6

BOOSTING YOUR ENERGY AND PHYSICAL PERFORMANCE

The chances are that your doctor has never seen a completely healthy person. Almost all medical research concerns itself only with ill people and disease. For this reason the world of athletics provides a unique chance to measure the effects of optimum nutrition on people who are supremely healthy.

For the athlete, excellent physical condition is the primary means to great achievements. Many top sportsmen and women follow special diets, take supplements[1] and keep extremely fit and healthy. I certainly didn't expect to find signs of sub-optimum vitamin deficiency among the athletes I tested, but to my surprise I did not find one without signs of nutritional deficiency. Since optimum nutrition improves the efficiency of muscle cells,[2] I wanted to test its effect on athletes, especially during endurance sports such as cycling or long-distance running.

Optimum Nutrition Improves Endurance

My first study was with a group of amateur racing cyclists.[3] Cycling, like long-distance running, is one of the harder endurance sports. I selected five cyclists, ranging from the ages of 19 to 48. Each had a series of nutritional tests to calculate his or her optimum requirements and was then given supplement programmes and dietary suggestions for a period of three months. Each was interviewed before and after by a nutritionist and a doctor. We monitored their best times over 25 miles before and after supplementation, and asked them to rate their own improvements subjectively in performance, recovery time and health problems.

Their change in times ranged from an improvement of 6.5 minutes at one end to a loss of almost one minute at the other! But only one of the six registered a poorer time after supplementation; the other five all showed gains. The average improvement over the six was more than 1.5 minutes, reducing the time taken from 60.5 minutes to just under 59 minutes.

The doctors' and cyclists' own comments are revealing. Here are some of them:

Doctors' reports: 'Feels more alert. Also thinks he sleeps better.' 'Recovery time after races is better.' 'Undoubtedly racing better. Feels less tired and more alert and positive.'

Cyclists' reports: 'I feel fresher, my times have improved.' 'My cycling performance is better and my recovery rate after races is tremendous.'

One of the cyclists even noted that after taking the vitamin supplements he was no longer allergic to coffee; another, a woman, experienced a marked improvement in the degree of premenstrual tension that she usually suffered.

My results confirmed the earlier findings of Dr Colgan, who had tested the effects of nutrition on marathon runners.[4] There is little doubt that optimum nutrition does improve endurance, although these findings are all very recent and need to be confirmed by further research. The effects of optimum nutrition would also be much more pronounced after six months to a year, than after only three months.

Good Nutrition Makes You Strong

What have Sylvester Stallone and Christopher Reeve got in common? They both take a careful balance of nutritional supplements to maintain their Goliath-like strength. Optimum nutrition has been shown to increase not only endurance, but also sheer muscle-power. The effect is best illustrated in a study by Dr Colgan in which four experienced weightlifters were split into two groups. One group was given a special supplement programme, the other placebos. After three months, those on supplements had increased the maximum weight they could lift by about 50 per cent. The others, on dummy tablets, had only a 10 to 20 per cent increase. During the following three months, the supplements and the placebos were swapped around. Those previously on placebos caught up with the other weightlifters.[5]

For us mere mortals, vitamins really do give us increased vitality and energy. Lack of energy should be considered a disease. More of my clients complain of flagging energy than of any other symptom. For example, when Liz L. first saw me she was exhausted after a 9 am to 4 pm job. 'My husband wouldn't talk to me till at least 6 pm. I was grumpy, exhausted and often fell asleep. Since being on the vitamin programme I'm able to work from 8 am to 5 pm and I come home feeling wide awake. My husband and I get on much better, too!'

Although measuring energy is difficult, we all know the difference between feeling vital and alive, or tired and lethargic. From my own experience with hundreds of clients, I know that increased energy is the first sign of improvement. Our last survey of clients showed that 73 per cent notice a definite improvement in energy after following our recommendations.[6] Increased energy is also reported by people who start doing regular physical exercise. Although we have a lot to learn about the chemistry of well-being, it is likely that this effect is partly due to an increased rate of metabolism and to the production of certain nerve-chemicals in the body. One group of chemicals, called endorphins,[7] are thought to act as natural 'highs', making us feel happy and alert. It is known that vitamin C increases the production of endorphins. So does exercise - and music! Now you know why joggers listening to personal stereos are always smiling!

Keeping a Healthy Heart

With cardiovascular disease being the number one killer in the west today, our attention is inevitably drawn to the role of nutrition and exercise. Both have been shown to help, but neither appears to provide all the answers. Jim Fixx, the famous author of 'The Complete Book of Running', died at the age of 52 from a heart attack while jogging. The autopsy found that two of his coronary arteries were almost totally clogged, which is not so surprising to those who knew of his disregard for dietary advice. On the other hand, the heart surgeon, Dr Albert Starr, an advocator of the low-cholesterol diet, needed open-heart surgery at only 47 years of age. Having performed the very same operation over 3,000 times, he had followed all the guidelines for staying free of heart disease.

Which is more important, diet or exercise? Bill Solomon from the University of Arizona designed an experiment to find out the answer.[8] He got some obliging pigs to run around a track, but fed them the average vitamin-deficient diet. Another group ate the pig-equivalent of health food but had no exercise; and a third group had both exercise and good nutrition. The third group of pigs fared best, proving that exercise and good nutrition together are vital for optimum health.

Your pulse rate is the simplest means to keep a check on the health of your strongest muscle, the heart. A fast resting pulse rate of 100 beats per minute reflects a weak heart, which has to beat frequently to keep your blood flowing through the arteries and veins. On the other hand, a resting pulse of 50 beats per minute, the average for good marathon runners, represents a heart that is twice as strong. The 'normal' pulse rate is set at 72 beats per minute, although for someone leading a sedate lifestyle a pulse of 65 would be nearer the ideal. The resting pulse rate should not go up substantially with age. For example, my pulse was 72 at the age of 18 and is now 60, with my exercise level remaining the same. This is consistent with the findings by other researchers on the effects of nutrition. One study found that the average pulse rate of 18 women dropped from 76 to 68 beats per minute after six months of optimum nutrition.[9]

While it used to be thought that the fatty deposits that cause the arteries to narrow were the results of excess cholesterol in the diet and hence in the blood, recent evidence suggests a different explanation. Arterial deposits form only in certain parts of the circulation system. It appears that the cells in the artery wall in these areas begin to over-multiply, a bit like cancer cells, and accumulate only certain kinds of damaged cholesterol. Both damage to cells and cholesterol is caused by 'free radicals', by-products of oxygen (these are explained in more detail in Chapter 7). Vitamins C and E and the mineral selenium help prevent free radical damage, and are therefore crucial additions in a diet for a healthy heart.[10]

Monitoring Your Blood Pressure

Your blood pressure is a measure of the health of your arteries. Every time your heart beats, the pressure in your arteries reaches a maximum. Then there is a lull before the next beat. The maximum pressure is your 'systolic' pressure and the minimum is your 'diastolic' pressure. These are written with the systolic pressure first, followed by the diastolic: for example, 120/80. Blood pressures greater than this example can indicate the beginnings of narrowing or hardening of the arteries. A blood pressure of 150/95 is getting serious. The old 'rule of thumb' of allowing your systolic blood pressure to be 100 plus your age (e.g. 160 if you are 60 years old) is inaccurate. With good nutrition and exercise, your blood pressure should reduce to below 130/90, considerably decreasing your risk of cardiovascular disease.

Since raised blood pressure is usually the result of the formation of deposits in the arteries over many years, it rarely comes down substantially even after six months of nutritional treatment. After four years, however, one group of men with a marginally high blood pressure of 140/90 had reduced this to 120/80 without any drugs or increase in exercise.[11] A level of 120/80 represents a very low risk of cardiovascular disease. However, blood levels of cholesterol and triglycerides, which are associated with high risk, have been shown to reduce substantially in as little as three months. Contrary to popular belief, the dietary intake of cholesterol has little to do with the level of cholesterol in the blood.[12] There is remarkably little substantial evidence to show that a diet low in fats, but high in cholesterol, is in any way associated with heart disease.[13] However, there is no doubt that reducing your intake of saturated fats can only be beneficial.

Supplements Decrease Blood Pressure

Many individual nutrients have been shown to lower high blood pressure and help maintain a healthy cardiovascular system. Among these are vitamins A, B3, B6, C and E and minerals calcium, magnesium, potassium, selenium, zinc, manganese and chromium. Also important are essential fatty acids, especially EPA. What would be the effect of supplementing all of these in combination? Three ION researchers selected 34 volunteers with mild to moderate hypertension and gave each a comprehensive multivitamin and mineral supplement programme over 12 weeks. During this time there was a steady and significant drop in blood pressure.[14]

7
INCREASING YOUR HEALTHY LIFESPAN

The quest for immortality or, at least, extended lifespan is nothing new. Since the beginning of history, myths and legends about magic potions and ancient men have abounded. But now, as we approach the twenty-first century, many scientists and gerontologists (gerontology is the study of ageing) are predicting that a lifespan of 120 will soon be possible. For some, extended lifespan means prolonged old age and more years of misery. For others, it is deemed unnatural or not 'the will of God'.

But ageing is not a function of time. Certainly they go together, but that does not mean that the passage of time causes one to age. After all, a 50-year-old man can have a biological age of 30 or 70. Why the difference? Nor are most deaths 'natural'. Over 75 per cent of deaths are caused by diseases like cancer, heart disease, bronchial infections or accidents. Would it not be preferable if we could live our entire and extended life in optimum health until the day we died?

What is the Maximum Lifespan?
To understand the science of life extension, many different questions must be asked. What is the known maximum achieved lifespan? What are the necessary conditions for living long? What happens when we age? What are the major causes of death, and can these be prevented? And lastly, how can we extend the maximum?

According to gerontologist Dr Walford, it is unlikely that anyone has lived beyond 120 years old.[1] Most claims for longevity cannot be proved beyond a doubt. For example, Attila the Hun (died 500 AD) was supposed to have lived to 121, and Jonathon Hartrop (died 1791), from the Yorkshire village of Aldbrough, was said to have attained the ripe old age of 138. However, birth and death records are simply not good enough to substantiate such claims. More recent records of the Hunzas, an Indian tribe, and inhabitants of the Caucasus in the USSR, are also likely to be exaggerations. For example, one villager was reported in the Soviet papers to be 130 - until his fellow villagers identified him as a deserter in World War I, who had used his father's papers to avoid being returned to the front. In fact, he was only 78. What fame is there in being an aged 78? But to be 130 immediately makes one noble, a celebrity. The oldest person with fully acceptable credentials was Izumi, a Japenese fisherman who died in 1986 at the age of 120. He was essentially healthy up to the age of 113. Fanny Thomas, from California, lived to be 113 years and 215 days and died in1980. She attributed her longevity to the fact that she ate apple sauce three times a day and never married, so "never had a man to bother me".' With the exception of the tortoise, which can live to be 150, human beings are the longest living animals.

What is the Average Lifespan?

Contrary to popular belief, there has been little change in the average lifespan in the last 60 years. At the bottom end of the scale, vast increases in general sanitation and preventative approaches to infectious and contagious diseases such as smallpox have dramatically improved our chances of survival early in life. But once we are aged 45, our average life expectancy is now 74 - in the 1920s it was 72. Few of us are still alive at the age of 100, and even fewer at 110. The major reasons for this is not infectious disease, but degenerative diseases such as cancer and cardiovascular diseases - and, of course, accidents.

How to Live Longer

The first major breakthrough in ageing has already begun: it is the decrease in deaths due to cardiovascular disease. Accounting for over 40 per cent of deaths in the 1970s but only 12 per cent in 1900, it is logical to assume that strokes (blockages in the arteries at the base of the head) and heart disease have come about through something we are doing that we were not doing 100 years ago. Along with a decline in overall fitness,[2] we now have increased consumption of sugar,[3] fat[4] and refined foods[5] (causing a lower intake of vitamins and minerals), increased smoking[6] and increased exposure to environmental pollution and chemicals in our food. Too often we accept the death of a relative or friend as an 'act of God' or bad luck. But there is virtually no element of chance involved in cardiovascular disease, which has now reached epidemic proportions. In the nineteenth century the same views were held about the contagious diseases until the causes for these were understood and later eradicated. And many of the factors listed above are also responsible for our increased rate of cancer.

Preventing the Major Killers with Optimum Nutrition

I have already mentioned the role of vitamins C and E and the mineral selenium in the prevention of heart disease; vitamins against cancer is my next concern. Cancer cells are cells that continue to divide and multiply, like our own cells do during development in the womb. This unruly cellular behaviour occurs either because environmental factors (carcinogens) damage the cell's internal behaviour code (its DNA), or due to errors of metabolism, sometimes the consequence of nutritional deficiency. Every day cancer cells are produced and begin to multiply, but fortunately we have an efficient 'hit squad' - the immune system. The cells of the immune system carry out 24-hour surveillance on these misfit cells and destroy them before it's too late. However, if the immune system isn't strong enough, the cancer cells keep multiplying and protect themselves from the immune system. A cell mass that doesn't spread is called a benign tumour. A tumour that continues to grow is called, depending on location, a carcinoma (if it is in epithelial tissue - the inner or outer skin of the body, such as lung or colon), sarcoma (if it is in supporting structures like fibrous tissue) and leukaemia (if it is in blood-forming cells) or lymphoma (if it is in lymph nodes). These are all forms of cancer.

With nutrition, we have three lines of defence. The first involves the prevention of DNA damage; the second, the strengthening of the immune system, and the third, the avoidance or neutralisation of carcinogens. One of the major causes of cell damage is the behaviour of free radicals. A free radical is an atom or group of atoms with an uneven electrical charge. To complete itself it steals a charged particle (an electron) from a neighbouring cell, which can set up a chain of reactions producing more free radicals, damaging more cells and causing them to misbehave. Many normal chemical reactions, such as breathing in oxygen, give rise to the formation of free radicals. These free radicals damage many cells, but most can effect repair. However, especially later in life, heart muscle cells, nerve and brain cells do not replace themselves so readily and are more permanently affected by damage. Unsaturated oils, which are found in cell membranes, are particularly susceptible to free radical damage. So we have developed ways of dealing with these by-products of using oxygen. These are anti-oxidants.

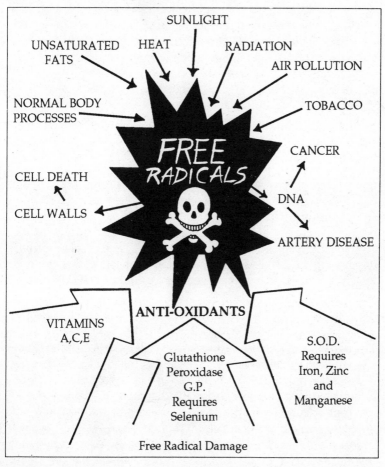

Figure 6 *Anti-Oxidant Nutrients and Sources of Free Oxidising Radicals*

Anti-oxidants, like vitamin C and vitamin E, protect our cells from free radical attack. Both have been shown to increase lifespan.[7] Nuts and seeds also contain vitamin E to protect their essential oils from oxidation, which is the same as rancidity. Yet some oil manufacturers remove vitamin E and sell us vegetable oil that is prone to rancidity.

We also have enzymes designed to disarm free radicals. One of these, SOD (superoxide dismutase), is at the forefront of both cancer and cardiovascular research, which has led to the sale of SOD tablets in health food shops. Yet there is little evidence that SOD taken in tablets can survive the perils of digestion and remain intact to strengthen us from the ageing effect of oxides. One type of SOD, however, which is dependent on the presence of manganese, may explain why supplements of manganese decrease the incidence of sarcoma cancers in rats.[8] Another SOD depends on a careful balance of copper and zinc. An excess of copper or a deficiency of zinc have also been shown to be associated with increased cancers.[9]

A close relative anti-oxidant enzyme, GP (glutathione peroxidase), depends on the mineral selenium. Increase the dietary intake of selenium by a factor of ten and you will double the activity of GP.[10] In both animals and man high selenium is associated with low risk of cancer. In one study 111 patients who developed cancer within a five-year period were compared to a control group of 210 people who remained cancer-free. The selenium level in the cancer victims was significantly lower. Those with very low selenium levels had double the chance of getting cancer compared to those with very high selenium levels. Also, parts of the world rich in selenium have typically low rates of breast cancer. On the basis of this evidence, which is supported by extensive animal studies, I take 100 mcg of selenium every day.

Strengthening the White Army

The immune system is like an army of cells, with a mission to seek out and destroy invaders. Invaders can be viruses, bacteria or cancer cells, all of which are recognised as alien. Our army consists of white blood cells that can be broken down into smaller units. These include macrophages, which gather round inflamed or infected areas and gobble up foreign particles, and lymphocytes. B-lymphocytes help produce antibodies that are specifically designed to destroy the invaders or antigens. Another type, called 'natural killer' lymphocytes, are particularly good at destroying cancer cells. Of course, these cells are themselves very destructive and their numbers must be controlled. T-lymphocytes are designed to do this job. But none of these works without an adequate supply of vitamins.[11]

To have maximum protection from infection, you need to be able to produce the antibodies specifically geared to the invading organism. This system forms the basis of inoculation: a small amount of 'flu virus, for example, enables your white army to produce its antibodies for defence next time. Deficiency of vitamins B2, B5 and B6 have all been shown to decrease antibody production.[12] Lymphocytes become less active when folic acid or B12 levels are low.[13] B vitamins support your white army, protecting you from cancer cells and strengthening you against viruses.

Detoxifying Carcinogens

Asbestos and cigarette smoke are well-known carcinogens, but there are more than 5,000 other substances known to promote cancer. Among these nitrosamines, nitrates and nitrites are particularly prevalent.[14] The worldwide use of artificial fertilizers has caused a massive increase in the amount of nitrates we consume in our food. If hydrochloric acid levels are low, or vitamin C absent, nitrates, in turn, can combine in the digestive tract to form the highly carcinogenic nitrosamines.[15] Low vitamin A levels are associated with a high risk of lung cancer and this has highlighted the role of vitamin A in protecting the 'inside skin' of the lungs and digestive tract from carcinogens.[16]

A three-pronged attack against cancer and ageing must involve nutrients to strengthen the immune system (vitamins B2, B5, B6 and B12; folic acid; vitamins A, C and E and zinc); nutrients to protect us from cellular damage (vitamins A, C and E, zinc, manganese and selenium), and nutrients to detoxify carcinogens (vitamins C and A).

Accidents and Ageing

In nature, far more deaths occur through accidents than from any other cause. The most common accident is getting eaten - one which we need fear no longer. Some organisms, such as sea anemones, do not age: their population is kept under control entirely through accidents. For mankind, accidents account for six per cent of all deaths, nearly half of these involving motor vehicles. This accident rate is more than double that at the beginning of the century and is probably the result of a changing physical environment, including a dramatic increase in deaths from road traffic accidents.

Once we've avoided the accidents, and prevented the degenerative diseases such as hardening of the arteries and cancer, why then do we age? One theory, known as the Hayflick limit, suggests that our cells are pre-programmed to self-destruct.17 Within the nucleus of each cell ticks away a timebomb; when time runs out, the cell dies. While a substantial amount of evidence supports this theory (for example, if you put a new nucleus in an old cell, the cell lives longer), it is unlikely that this explanation is the whole story.

A brilliant piece of research suggested another mechanism, based on the rate of repair of our 'blueprint for survival', the DNA molecule.18 The DNA molecule contains the information to build new and healthy cells. Since we build some billions of cells every day, the accuracy of our DNA is crucial. Yet DNA is itself often damaged by normal chemical reactions in the body, as well as by radiation, cigarette smoke and other environmental pollutants. By comparing the rate of repair of DNA in different species of animals, the researchers found that those which repaired DNA most rapidly lived longest. Since one of the principal causes of DNA damage is the action of free radicals, anti-oxidants like vitamins C and E are seen to be essential for a healthy lifespan.

DrJames Fleming at the Linus Pauling Institute of Science and Medicine has found that the lifespan of all species relates, more or less, to a fixed number of heart beats - around 2.5 billion. This suggests that keeping the heart strong and healthy is a key factor.

Another sign of ageing is a weakened immune system. The immune system is designed to recognise anything that is not 'us' and destroy it. For example, when we are exposed to a virus, the immune system is activated to produce macrophages and lymphocytes, which attach to and gobble up the invading virus. As we age, our immune system weakens. With that, the ability to fight off infections and keep cancer cells at bay declines. With more than 17 per cent of deaths coming from cancer, and nearly 4 per cent from pneumonia, 'flu or bronchial infections, strengthening the immune system is vital.

But the immune system doesn't always go wrong by becoming bad at its job. Sometimes it attacks itself. SLE (systemic lupus erythematosus), an auto-immune disease, serves as a good example of a disease in which the victim produces anti-bodies that destroy its own cells. Optimum nutrition can help here as well. My first client with SLE was under close medical surveillance because she produced so many self destructive antibodies. After 12 months of optimum nutrition her antibody count had dropped dramatically and all her symptoms were gone.

Many diseases whose symptoms include signs of rapid ageing show the same auto-immune response. Perhaps our cellular pacemaker is programmed to end life through this form of self-destruction. Salmon do something like it, using hormones. After four years in the open sea, salmon find their way back to the place where they were born where, after spawning, their adrenal glands release a massive amount of hormones. The fish age within minutes to the point of death.

Examination of the various theories of ageing shows that a possible human lifespan of more than 100 years is far from an illusion. By making healthy cells, preventing and repairing DNA damage, and optimising the health of your immune system, lifespan can be pushed to the limits.

Eat Less and Live Longer

Improving our nutrition isn't the only thing we can do to stay young. Exercise and undernutrition are also important keys. A 300 per cent increase in lifespan through calorie restriction has been found in fish,[19] and a 60 per cent increase in rats.[20] Calorie restriction - undernutrition - is not the same as malnutrition. The evidence is clear: keep the calories low, but the quality of nutrition high. These studies, involving severe calorie restriction, have not been carried out on man for obvious ethical reasons.[21] Yet it is more than likely that the leaner you are the longer you'll live. With today's diet that means low fat and sugar and extra vitamin supplements. But be careful. Crash diets are especially inadvisable and are not the best way to live longer, or to lose weight (see chapter 11). Calorie reduction should be a very gradual process. Many of my clients in fact lose weight on optimum nutrition programmes without even trying, because optimum nutrition leaves one craving less and eating less.

Exercise Keeps You Young

Regular exercise can add seven years to your lifespan, concludes Drs Rose and Cohen of the Veterans' Administration Hospital in Boston. But the exercise must be continued late in life and must be 'aerobic' - i.e. your heart rate must reach 80 per cent of its maximum for at least twenty minutes. Cycling, swimming, brisk walking and running are good; on the other hand, weightlifting, yoga and strengthening exercises do little to extend your life. Aerobic exercise reduces blood cholesterol levels,[22] pulse and blood pressure, promoting better cardiovascular health as well as increasing mental function. It also helps you to maintain proper blood sugar control thereby especially helping diabetics.[23]

The Not too Distant Future

No one knows for sure what breakthrough in life extension will occur in the next 30 years. But given what we know now, lifespan can be extended by at least ten years through optimum nutrition, even if you start late in life. The experts are certainly optimistic.

"Provided you are not in the grip of a degenerative disease already, you are likely to get at least a decade of vigorous years, and perhaps a lot more, added to your life, no matter what age you are now," says Dr Michael Colgan. "It seems fairly certain that maximum lifespan could already be prolonged to 130 or 140 years by the exercise of very stringent measures," says Dr Roy Walford, leading gerontologist. Nobel prize winner Dr Linus Pauling, aged 91, believes that optimum nutrition with extra vitamin C could add 16 to 24 years to the average lifespan.

"The long-term effects of optimum nutrition are at least an extra ten years of healthful living," said Dr Carl Pfeiffer, who had a massive heart attack at 51 and was given a maximum of ten years to live - if he had a pacemaker fitted. Instead, he pursued optimum nutrition, taking 10g of vitamin C a day. He outlived his four brothers and sisters and was working an energetic 14 hours a day right up to the last week of his life, which ended at the age of 80.

Dr Roger Williams, who died at the age of 95, sometimes called the father of optimum nutrition, said "Well-rounded nutrition, including generous amounts of vitamins C and E, can contribute materially to extending the healthy lifespan of those who are already middle-aged. The greatest hope for increasing lifespans can be offered if nutrition - from the time of prenatal development to old age - is continuously of the highest quality."

8

STRENGTHENING YOUR IMMUNE SYSTEM

The immune system consists of a collection of special cells that move around in the blood and lymphatic system, an army on a 24 hour 'search and destroy' mission. They look for alien invaders, whether rogue cells, viruses, bacteria or substances that we are allergic to. These special cells travel between the cells of our body, but are mainly concentrated in our network of lymphatic vessels. They drain into lymph glands, concentrated in the neck, armpit and groin, and from there lead into the central lymphatic system where our immune army is strongest.

Once an intruder has found its way inside the body our immune army is alerted. It's troops consist of many different battalions of blood cells. These include special "scout" cells that squeeze in and out of blood vessel walls on the lookout for trouble. Once they find an invader they attempt to engulf it. If they have difficulty they summon up more troops called T-lymphocytes. These ingest any invader they come across. To keep them in check there are T-suppressor cells, that 'turn them off', and T-helper cells that 'turn them on'. (The AIDS virus, for example, selectively destroys T-helper cells which leads to a relative excess of the T-suppressor cells and to an eventual weakening of the immune system.)

Perhaps even more important than T-lymphocytes are B-lymphocytes. These cells have the ability to produce tailor made antibodies that stop the invader dead in its tracks. So if you have an allergy to milk, the B lymphocytes will produce hundreds of thousands of antibodies seconds after you drink milk. It was the discovery of this, the body's ability to produce a specific weapon to deal with each invader, that led to the development of immunisation.

When a battle is raging between your blood cells and an invader, the body turns up the temperature which helps the immune cells to fight. A high temperature and swollen lymph glands are the classic signs of infection, coupled with the effects of the particular virus - a sore throat, for example, or nausea and diarrhoea. The consequences are familiar to us all. Headache, excessive mucus production and coughing are just some of the symptoms of a viral or bacterial attack.

If it's any consolation, the worse the symptoms, the harder your system is fighting.

Strengthening Your Defences

By keeping your body's guard up, you can win the war against invaders before the battle has even begun. You have three strategies at your disposal. Firstly you need strong cell walls to keep out invaders, including viruses and bacteria; secondly you need to maintain a stout army of immune cells with healthy production of new immune cells; and thirdly you need to be armed against the weapons of free radicals.

Your first line of defence is the skin, including the 'inside skin' which lines the lungs and digestive system. Many viruses, for example hepatitis and the AIDS virus, cannot cross the skin barrier and need to enter the body via fluids. Even carcinogens - substance that are thought to induce cancer, of which cigarette smoke is an example - are less likely to do damage if your first line of defence is strong. This strength depends upon maintaining the integrity of your cell walls. To keep your cell walls strong, you must maintain your level of vitamin A. Carrots and other orange-yellow foods like tomatoes, beetroot and apricots are rich in this vital vitamin. So are liver, kidneys and cashew nuts. Children need more vitamin A than adults because it stimulates growth and the maturing of the immune system.

Calcium and magnesium are also important for strong cells and a healthy immune army. These are particularly needed by the elderly and particularly by post menopausal women whose decline in oestrogen production means that calcium is poorly absorbed. Dairy products, while rich in calcium, are a poor source of magnesium. Only green leafy vegetables, nuts and seeds provide these essential elements.

Vitamin C is important too. It increases the production of T-lymphocyte cells and helps produce antibodies and improve their performance.[1] Vitamin C is also a crucial weapon, along with vitamins A and E, in your defence against free radical attack.

Free Radical Attack

Many viruses try to force an entry into our cells. Cancer cells go one step further and try to destroy neighbouring cells and take over their space. This is done by releasing a barrage of toxic and other substances, including 'free radicals'. Free radicals are atoms, or groups of atoms, with an uneven electrical charge. Because they are uneven they try to balance themselves by stealing an electron from a neighbour. The easiest electrons to steal are from essential fats that form part of every single cell wall which then becomes weakened, making it easier for invading toxins, bacteria and viruses to get in. Free radicals are also created by eating fried foods, from pollution and smoking.

But nature has devised specific protectors, called anti-oxidants, that help to mop up these enemies. They are vitamins A, C and E - most of all vitamin E because it is a fat soluble vitamin designed to protect fats. All natural foods rich in polyunsaturated fats and oils are also rich in vitamin E. But as we process these oils, for example in cooking, the vitamin E is destroyed and the oil left open to free radical attack. So adequate vitamin E is another requirement for keeping our cell walls intact. One mineral, selenium, helps complete our defence against free radicals. Although needed in tiny amounts of 50 mcg a day (less than a millionth of our daily requirement of protein) it is no less important.

How To Boost Your Immune Power

So what can you do to boost your immune power? The answer is a lot. Many factors are involved in keeping your immune system working well. Getting plenty of light stimulates the thymus, and exercise stimulates movement of lymph and boosts the immune system. Stress causes the release of a hormone called cortisol, which is a powerful suppressor of the immune system. Pollution can overload the body's defences, so it is best to avoid additives and eat organic food where possible. Ensuring that you get a good nights sleep is also important to keep your immune system in good shape.

Diet is perhaps the most important factor. Fat and fat soluble vitamins are transported in the lymph, so a diet high in fat makes the lymph thicker and less mobile. Some nutritionists think that an excess of dairy produce which is particularly mucus forming, also clogs up the lymph. Fried food is doubly bad because it is both high in fat and free radicals that damage and weaken body cells.

Getting enough protein in your diet is important. Fish, chicken, beans and lentils are good sources of protein. While eating less fat and getting enough protein are not too difficult, few people get enough immune boosting vitamins and minerals from their diet. Vitamins and minerals are vital for immune power. Many of the B vitamins, including B5 (pantothenic acid), B6, B12 and folic acid are needed to produce immune cells.[2] In severe B6 deficiency no antibodies are produced at all![3] B vitamins are found in fresh vegetables, grains, nuts and seeds.

Vitamin C is the most important of all. It helps to knock out viruses by increasing T-lymphocyte production. It destroys many bacteria. It helps produce antibodies and seems to improve their performance. It also helps to relieve the symptoms of sore eyes and runny nose because it is a natural antihistamine. All fruit, but especially oranges and kiwis are rich in vitamin C. So are red peppers. Vitamins A and E are both anti-oxidants protecting cells from damage. Vitamin A also strengthens cell walls, keeping invaders out.

Of the minerals, calcium, magnesium, selenium and zinc are the most important. According to Dr. Stephen Davies, "zinc has a profound effect on the immune system responses. When zinc is deficient, children become prone to infections".[4]

Zinc increases T-lymphocyte production, the cells that destroy alien invaders, and helps the thymus gland, the cornerstone of the immune system, to work.[5] Although immune cells are produced in different parts of the body, mainly in the bone marrow, T-lymphocytes only become mature in the thymus gland in the chest. From puberty onwards the thymus shrinks and may be only a quarter of its original size by the time you are 50. It used to be thought that this was normal, but increasingly scientists are considering that it may be the result of zinc and vitamin A deficiency. In one study involving people with known zinc deficiency, the thymus actually grew in size after only ten days of zinc supplementation.[6]

Winning the Cold War
There are basically two methods of defence against colds. The first

is to prevent infection in the first place. The second is to minimise the effect of infection once it occurs. Cold viruses are not technically 'alive' as they cannot reproduce. They can only multiply if they get inside your cells and get these invaded cells to make more virus particles. In order to keep viruses out you need to have sufficient vitamin A in your body and enough calcium and magnesium to make those cell walls strong enough to resist the virus.

At the onset of winter, the external temperature gets colder and the body becomes less able to use its supply of vitamin A. This starts a vicious circle with vitamin A becoming more and more in demand. This is probably one of the reasons why zinc is helpful when you've got a cold because it allows vitamin A, stored in the liver, to be used.

The secret of any battle is to be well prepared. Start by making sure that you have adequate nutrients to keep your immune system at the ready. Your multivitamin supplement should contain at least 7,500 iu of vitamin A and at least 1,000mg of vitamin C as well as a good B complex (one which contains choline, pantothenate and folic acid). Your multimineral should contain zinc but not copper and at least half as much magnesium as calcium. If you're a person who often suffers from infections you may need to experiment with a maintenance dose of up to 20,000 ius of beta-carotene, which is a non-toxic form of vitamin A, and an additional 3 grams of vitamin C.

Is Your Early Warning System on Alert?

As with any attack the element of surprise gives a distinct advantage and unfortunately it is usually in the favour of the attacking virus. How do you know when you are under attack? Obviously, it is wise to be suspicious if you've been in the company of someone with a cold. Symptoms usually start two or three days after exposure. You also have your own 'early warning system' that tells you you have unwelcome guests. The warning signs are a sensation in the throat or nose on waking, a thick head or a hint of a headache, heavy muscles, feeling slightly tired even before you get up or feeling hot, cold or shaky. If you feel these symptoms don't hesitate to reach for the vitamin C. Even if it turns out to be a false alarm you can only benefit.

Why Enough Vitamin C is Essential

So many proper research trials have shown that large amounts of vitamin C lessen the frequency, shorten the duration and lessen the symptoms of a cold.[7] A recent review of sixteen such studies showed that, on average, 34 per cent less days of illness are experienced by those who supplement vitamin C.[8] So why do so many doctors still sneeze at vitamin C for colds? There are an equal number of papers that show no effect. However, a close look at these papers shows two common fundamental flaws. In some studies laboratory bred viruses are squirted up the poor subject's nose. These viruses are so virulent it's little wonder vitamin C shows no effect. It's a bit like testing a boxer's mouthguard by hitting him in the face with a sledgehammer! The more frequent blunder is a failure to administer enough vitamin C. The best results have been achieved using between 400mg and 1,000mg per hour. According to Dr.Linus Pauling "The amount of protection increases with increase in the amount of ingested vitamin C and becomes nearly complete with 10g to 40g per day taken at the immediate onset of a cold."[9] In fact, the amount needed depends very much on the person. A good policy is to take 3g immediately and 2g every four hours until symptoms subside which should be within 24 hours. Before going to bed take a further 3g. Although you can lessen the dose on subsequent days it is definitely wise to keep supplementing more than usual vitamin C for two days after symptoms have stopped. Stopping vitamin C suddenly can result in a return of symptoms. You may experience loose bowels on these large amounts, which is quite harmless, but that is all. There is no harm from taking large amounts of vitamin C for a few days.

In the long-term supplementing 1 to 3g of vitamin C every day helps to keep your immune system strong. It is probably best to supplement this with other nutrients needed to maintain a healthy immune system. One such supplement, Immunade, which provides vitamin A,E, zinc, selenium, calcium, magnesium and molybdenum as well as 1g of vitamin C, was tested in a double-blind trial at ION involving 37 people. After twelve weeks 81 per cent of those taking Immunade considered themselves less susceptible to colds, compared to 44 per cent on a placebo tablet.[10] The incidence of cold symptoms and the duration of symptoms were also considerably reduced in the Immunade group.

Seven Ways To Stop a Cold Dead in Its Tracks

1 Take 3 grams of vitamin C immediately and then two grams every four hours (or three times a day). Alternatively, mix 6 grams of vitamin C powder in fruit juice diluted with water and drink throughout the day. Some people prefer to use calcium ascorbate, a

less acidic form of vitamin C.

2 Also supplement other immune boosting nutrients, especially vitamins A and E, selenium, zinc.

3 Eat lightly, preferably relying mainly on fruits and vegetables, including foods rich in vitamins A and C, for example carrots, beetroot, green peppers and citrus fruit.

4 Avoid mucus forming and fatty foods, i.e. meat, eggs and milk produce. These make your lymphatic fluid thick, which is the main transport system for immune cells which carry invading viruses to lymph nodes for further punishment.

5 Avoid all alcohol, cigarettes, tea and coffee. Drink plenty of water and herb teas.

6 Take it easy. Do everything slowly and avoid stressful situations. Get some rest and plenty of sleep.

7 Once you think you've won, wait at least 24 hours then cut the vitamins down to 1 gram of vitamin C three times a day, and one immune boosting vitamin and mineral supplement in the morning. Once you have been well for three days go back to your normal supplement programme.

Understanding Allergies

The vast majority of people develop allergic reactions to foods or substances in the environment. What this means is that their immune systems have become sensitised to the substance, called an allergen, and launch an attack as if it were an invader. But what makes us allergic in the first place? We are designed to take in to the blood stream only digested foods, in other words simple carbohydrates, essential fatty acids and amino acids, not whole protein. If, for some reason our digestive processes are not working so well, or the gastrointestinal wall is 'leaky' we may take in whole proteins which the immune army will attack. Another reason for potential reactions is that the immune army is malnourished and hence over-reacts to innocuous substances. Allergies are therefore much more likely to develop in those that have a weakened immune system or poor digestion. The likely allergens are foods eaten frequently, especially those that are often introduced too early in infancy, are themselves gastrointestinal irritants, or are relatively new foods for the human organism.

   Wheat, for example, is eaten by most people every day. It contains a gastrointestinal irritant called gliadin which is part of wheat gluten. Grains are also a relatively recent addition to our diet. I recommend introducing wheat to infants late in the weaning process since it is Britain's number one allergen. On the other hand, an allergic reaction to vegetables is very rare.

So how do you know if you've got an allergy and, if you have, what can you do about it? In truth it is not easy to know what you're allergic to. Any good nutritionist will investigate your allergic potential by looking at your diet and the kind of symptoms you have. If necessary they can run tests to check for allergies but no tests are one hundred percent accurate.The best test is to avoid suspect foods and see how you feel. Once you know what you're reacting to the best strategy is to avoid these substances for at least three months and meanwhile build up your immune system through a proper supplement programme. Once optimally nourished many people can tolerate small amounts of substances they used to react to.

Overcoming Hayfever

Many hayfever sufferers are high histamine producers. This is particularly probable if there is a family history of hayfever since the over-production of histamine appears to be a genetic trait. We all store histamine within white blood cells, which is released during an allergic reaction. Those that over-produce histamine react more strongly. Vitamin C in doses of 3,000mg and more, and the combination of l-methionine 1,000mg and calcium 500mg helps to keep histamine under control, reducing allergic potential.[11] Vitamin B3, in the form of niacin, causes blushing, which is partly to do with the release of histamine. By releasing histamine, niacin can reduce the allergic potential of high histamine producers. They often experience a pronounced blushing effect the first few times, which normally lasts up to 30 minutes, with future supplementation failing to produce a similar effect. This is usually an indication that their histamine status has normalised.

The three most common allergens are wheat and grains, pollens, and dairy produce. Obviously grains and manypollens are products of the grass family. It is interesting to me that milk is produced by animals whose diet is exclusively grasses. I don't know if this connection has any significance. What I do know is that hayfever sufferers are much less likely to react if they avoid or reduce their intake of wheat, other grains and dairy produce.

One of the body's primary mechanisms for dealing with any inflammatory reaction is the anti-inflammatory function of the corticosteroids, hormones of the adrenal cortex. The production of corticosteroids depends upon an adequate supply of pantothenic acid. Supplementing between 250 and 750mg can reduce hayfever reactions considerably.

All of these measures are more likely to make a difference in people who have overall good nutrition, are not excessively stressed or suffering from other debilitating diseases. They are also more effective if started before the hayfever season. During periods of high pollen counts these supplements should be taken in the morning to provide protection during the day. Every hayfever reaction weakens one's resistance and therefore more effort is required to treat on-going hayfever than to encourage its prevention in susceptible individuals.

9
PROTECTING AGAINST POLLUTION

According to top British authorities, if we continue to pollute our environment the world will become irreversibly damaged within 50 years and inevitably unable to support life. Russian authorities are less optimistic and give us 15 years before its too late. As the battle to conserve our environment gains momentum, each one of us has a personal battle - to protect ourselves from pollution. In one year the average person breathes in two grams of solid pollution, eats 12 lbs of food additives, has up to a gallon of pesticides and herbicides spray on the fruits and vegetables they eat, receives nitrates, hormone and antibiotic residues both from water and food. No less than 6,000 new chemicals have been introduced into our food, our homes and the world around us in the last decade alone. These and other pollutants add to the burden our bodies already have to cope with from self-selected harmful substances including alcohol, cigarettes, recreational and medical drugs, free radicals from frying food, methylxanthines in coffee, and a host of naturally occurring toxins present in small amounts even in healthy food.

Although we are equipped with clever mechanisms for detoxifying harmful substances for many of us those mechanisms are becoming increasingly overloaded. When the total body burden of pollutants exceeds our ability to detoxify these substances are integrated into bone, fat, brain and other tissue. When calcium is released for normal body functions, so are toxins. When fat is used for energy, more toxins are released into the blood. Toxins that ultimately affect our brains, nervous system, liver, kidneys and other vital organs.

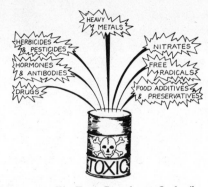

Figure 7 *The Toxic Barrel, our Cocktail of Pollutants*

The effects of pollution are cumulative and are rarely seen at the time the pollution occurs. It is not easy to link cause and effect between pollution-related diseases, when the pollution may have been slight over decades, or have occurred decades earlier. The origination of most diseases are themselves multifactorial. What we can be pretty certain of are the following negative effects:

Increased lead exposure causes a measurable decline in intelligence, performance and behaviour in the majority of children and a minority of adults.[1]

The level of nitrites and nitrates in most water supplies significantly increases the risk of certain forms of cancer.[2]

The level of free oxidising radicals, both from our polluted air, fried and processed foods, passive smoking and exhaust fumes, coupled with a deficiency in anti-oxidant nutrients, significantly weakens our immune system and increases our risk for most forms of cancer and heart disease.[3]

Long term ingestion of small amounts of aluminium from water, cooking utensils and food packaging is associated with premature senility.[4]

The reason why 30 per cent of pregnancies end in miscarriage, and 15 per cent of all babies born have physical defects, both of which are on the increase, is in part the result of increased pollution levels.[5]

These alarming facts represent the tip of the iceberg. Other diseases that have been associated with a high level of pollutants include all forms of arthritis, candidiasis, M.E. (post-viral syndrome), hyperactivity, high blood pressure, asthma, acne, eczema and schizophrenia. 'Minor' symptoms associated with increased body burden of pollutants include lethargy, drowsiness, mood swings, inability to concentrate, intolerance of fat or alcohol, poor skin, body odour, headaches, nausea, skin rashes, frequent infections and multiple allergies. All of these symptoms can occur for other reasons, such as specific diseases or deficiency in certain essential nutrients.

Even when these are the result of increased body pollution they are far more likely to occur in those who are not adequately nourished. This is because most pollutants are anti-nutrients, which means that they do their damage by interfering with the absorption or utilisation of nutrients, or by promoting their excretion. Lead, for example, interferes with calcium and zinc. Many of the symptoms of calcium and zinc deficiency are the same as the symptoms of too much lead. What's more, the body's detoxifying mechanisms are themselves greatly enhanced by an optimum intake of essential nutrients, including vitamins, minerals, essential fatty acids and protein.

Pollution Solutions

So how do you protect yourself from pollution? The first step is obvious. Avoid or reduce as much as possible your intake of pollutants. In case, by now you're suffering from 'acute pollution paranoia' console yourself with the fact that you cannot avoid all pollution. Harmful substances have always existed, even within foods whose overall effect on the body is definitely positive. The best we can do is minimise our overall exposure. One way to minimise our exposure is to increase the intake in our diet of certain factors that minimise the absorption of pollutants. The absorption of excess copper, for example, is minimised by the presence of zinc. Nitrites are less likely to form the cancer producing compounds nitrosamines, which are made in the digestive tract, when vitamin C is present.

The second step is to boost our natural mechanisms for detoxifying ourselves. This can be done using diet, supplements, internal cleansing and special breathing exercises. So let's now look at the major classes of pollutants, how to avoid or reduce our exposure to them, and how to protect ourselves from their harmful effects.

HEAVY METALS

Ourselves and our world are made out of elements. Many elements, like oxygen, calcium or zinc are essential, while other heavier elements, are not. The most common toxic elements are lead, aluminium, cadmium, mercury and arsenic in that order. Copper is also toxic in excess, but in small amounts it is essential.

We receive lead from air we breathe, the food we eat and the water we drink. The main source of lead is from fumes from leaded petrol. This air-borne lead ends up in the soil and on plants which we then eat. There is nowhere in Britain that is not polluted by lead. Even the level of lead in Greenland ice is a thousand times higher now compared to a hundred years ago.[6] Lead affects the brain in many ways. It interferes with neurotransmitters, making the brain more excitable. This results in hyperactivity and aggressive behaviour. In the developing brain nerves send out branches that connect with other nerves. Like the branches of a tree this process is called arborisation. In animals with elevated lead, 10 per cent less connections are formed. Children with high lead levels are also less intelligent.

Another element associated with mental retardation and behavioural problems is cadmium. The discovery of high levels of cadmium in smokers provides another reason to stop. Professor Bryce-Smith from Reading University demonstrated the damaging effects of these elements in an extraordinary piece of research. He analysed element levels in the placenta of 'normal' mothers, immediately after birth. He was able to predict both the birthweight of the newborn babies and their head circumference (a factor associated with mental retardation) from the levels of lead, cadmium and zinc. The higher the lead and cadmium levels and the lower the zinc in the mother, the lower the birth weight and head circumference![7]

Aluminium is impossible to avoid completely. It is so widely used in food packaging, cooking utensils, even in toothpaste, antacid medications, some cheese and infant milk formulas. Aluminium deposits in the brain and is hard to get rid of. Aluminium excess is associated with early memory loss and Alzheimer's disease, a form of senile dementia.[8] In Alzheimer's disease abnormal clusters of nerves appear in the brain. These have been shown to be very high in aluminium. The connection between accumulating aluminium and memory loss is strong.

Human body copper levels have increased substantially in the last hundred years due to its presence in water as a result of copper water pipes. The contraceptive pill also encourages the body's retention of copper. Copper is a strong zinc antagonist, so those with poor zinc status are more susceptible to the effects of excess copper.

AVOID

- Avoid buying unwrapped fruit and vegetables exposed to street traffic that do not require peeling.
- Wash all fruit and vegetables, preferably in a bowl of water with two tablespoons of vinegar added. This acidifies the water

and helps remove heavy metals.
- Discard the outer leaves of cabbage, lettuce etc.
- Drink filtered or bottled water.
- Be wary of eating fish caught off the British coast. It is said that frozen fish is caught in the further reaches of the North Sea and Arctic ocean. Limit your fish intake when you don't know the source and certainly avoid local shellfish or a Dover sole from Dover.
- Do not exercise by busy roads. In cities, the lead level is highest during overcast days, and lowest on a clear day after rain.
- Avoid multivitamin and mineral supplements containing copper unless the supplement containing ten times as much zinc as copper.
- Don't smoke and, where possible, avoid passive smoking.
- Avoid foods packaged in aluminium. Don't grill foods on, or wrap foods in aluminium foil.
- Don't take antacid medication containing aluminium.
- Don't use aluminium pots and pans. Many non-stick pans are aluminium once you've worn through the non-stick bit, which incidentally is toxic.

PROTECT
- Make sure your diet provides plenty of calcium, zinc and vitamin C, which are heavy metal antagonists. That means eating lots of nuts, seeds, green leafy vegetables, wheatgerm, fresh fruit etc.
- Eat foods high in pectin, which is also protective. This includes apples, bananas, carrots.
- Minimise alcohol, which increases the absorption of lead.
- Supplement your diet with at least 1,000mg of vitamin C, 200mg of calcium and 10mg of zinc. Double this amount if you live in a city. Magnesium (100mg) is also protective against aluminium toxicity, and selenium (100mcg) against arsenic and mercury toxicity.

DRUGS

As a nation , our consumption of medical drugs is the highest in the world. The British pharmaceutical industry turns over a staggering £2,000 million a year. But do we really need to take so many? The answer is no. For example, the use of aspirin for mild pain and headaches can never do us any long term good. The human body has no need for its active ingredient 'salicylic acid'. Continual use of aspirin is known to increase risk of stomach ulceration and kidney disease, as well as blocking vitamin C uptake and lowering folic acid levels. In 1980 the sixth World Nutrition Congress reported that even a single aspirin can cause intestinal bleeding for one week. The daily use of low doses of aspirin to thin the blood and protect against heart disease warrants extreme caution.

Some people take caffeine-based pain killers, since coffee drinkers deprived of coffee will suffer headaches as a sign of withdrawal. Out of the frying pan into the fire!

Another common and extremely dangerous drug is cortisone and cortisone like drugs. Cortisone is a synthetic form of the hormone produced by the adrenal gland to combat stress. This substance has almost magical qualities in that it can reduce pain, stop inflammatory reactions, prevent transplanted organs being rejected, and is now being used to treat over 100 different ailments including cancer, arthritis, kidney disease, hay fever and allergies. In America 29 million prescriptions for it are written each year! "The sad truth is that cortisone doesn't cure anything: it merely suppresses the symptoms of the disease" says Dr. Zumoff, formerly with the Steroid Research Laboratory at New York's Montefiore Hospital. One of the major problems with this class of drug is that the body stops producing its own cortisone. Wherever possible drugs are best avoided.

AVOID

- Avoid excessive use of pain killers.
- Avoid antacids containing aluminium.
- Avoid frequent use of antibiotics.
- Avoid anti-inflammatory drugs, both non-steroidal and steroid based medication.
- Avoid the use of anti-depressants and sleeping pills as much as possible.
- Investigate natural and barrier methods of birth control rather than taking the pill.

   Do not stop or reduce any prescribed medication without first consulting your doctor.

PROTECT

• If you take pain killers regularly increase your vitamin C intake by 1,000mg.

• If you are doing a course of antibiotics take a high strength B complex during the course, and supplement beneficial bacteria for two weeks after the course to recolonise your digestive tract with healthy bacteria.

• If you are on the pill take a high strength B complex and extra B6 to provide 100mg a day, plus zinc 15mg.

• If you take sleeping pills or anti-depressants also take a high strength B Complex (except in the case of MAOI anti-depressants such as Nardil or Parstelin in which case any source of yeast is best avoided.). Sleeping pills can often be replaced by l-tryptophan in doses of 1 to 3 grams.

NITRATES

Governments and the World Health Organisation have known for many years that nitrates and nitrites are toxic, and they set limits for water and food levels in 1970. Once inside the body nitrates combine with amines, present in almost all foods, to form nitrosamines, which are highly carcinogenic (cancer-producing) compounds. Most water authorities do not have the necessary purification equipment and consequently millions of people in Britain are consuming water containing nitrates at a level above the EEC top limit. The problem is especially severe in arable areas and the Thames basin, since nitrates, originating from use in fertilisers, have filtered down into the water table. The only way to solve this problem is to stop using nitrate based fertilisers and switch to organic farming methods.

Nitrates are consequently high in vegetables grown with nitrate based fertilisers, as well as water. Nitrates are also added to cured meats such as ham, sausages, bacon and pies. 70% of our intake comes from vegetables, 21% from water and 6% from meat.[8]

AVOID

• Drink filtered or bottled water.

• Eat organically grown produce wherever possible.

• Brush and floss your teeth regularly. It is estimated that up to 65% of nitrites absorbed are produced in the mouth by bacteria.

• Avoid foods that include nitrates or nitrites as preservatives, which includes many meat products.
• Make sure your protein intake is adequate, not excessive.

PROTECT

• Supplement your diet with at least 1,000mg of vitamin C. This inhibits nitrosamine formation. It is best to take some vitamin C with each meal. Glycine and vitamin E also have protective effects.
• If you suspect you do not produce enough stomach acid, for example, you do not digest foods well or feel nourished from the food you eat and are prone to flatulence, take a digestive enzyme formula containing hydrochloric acid, since a lack of hydrochloric acid enhances the formation of nitrosamines.

PESTICIDES

With today's chemical farming even the old adage that 'an apple a day keeps the doctor away' must be questioned. For the caterpillar, one brief journey across the average apple is enough to kill it. But what about us? In 1984 over 3,000 incidents of illness resulting from pesticide poisoning were recorded - including one death.

A survey by the Minister of Agriculture, Food and Fisheries found that between 89% and 99% of all fresh fruit, cereals and vegetables is sprayed with pesticides.[9] That also means that most meat and milk is contaminated from pesticides used in the animal's food. Although few proper surveys have been carried out to find the size of the problem, the Association for Public Analysts is gravely concerned. The association randomly tested 305 fruits. 31 of these samples contained levels of pesticides above the levels deemed safe, and a further 72 samples showed lower pesticide levels. Some fruits particularly strawberries , raspberries, grapes and tomatoes had measurable levels of at least six different pesticides![10]

AVOID

• Select organic fruit and vegetables wherever possible.
• Wash or peel non-organic produce.
• Choose fruits and vegetables in season. This means that your exposure to the chemicals used to delay ripening, prolong shelf

life, preserve colour and so on, will be limited.

PROTECT
• Supplement your diet with anti-oxidant nutrients, that's vitamins A, C and E and the minerals zinc and selenium since the detoxification of many pesticides involve these nutrients.

FOOD ADDITIVES

A number of chemicals are purposely added to our food to change its colour, preserve it longer, prevent rancidity, keep fats emulsified and foods stable. Most of them are synthetic compounds, some with known negative health effects. But the important point is that we really don't know what the long-term consequences of consuming relatively large amounts of additives is. It is therefore best to avoid all additives with a few notable exceptions.

AVOID
• Avoid all foods containing additives except...
• The colours E101(Vitamin B2), E160 (carotene, vitamin A)
• The anti-oxidants E300-304 (Vitamin C), E306-309 (Tocopherols, like vitamin E)
• The emulsifier E322 (lecithin)
• Stabilisers E375 (Niacin), E440 (Pectin)

PROTECT
• Since foods without preservatives are more likely to go off, it's important to buy fresh produce and consume it relatively quickly.

FREE RADICALS

Probably the single greatest cause of ill-health is free oxidising radicals. These are incomplete molecules containing oxygen which have an uneven electrical charge. All stable atoms and collections of atoms, called molecules, have an even electrical charge. Free radicals don't, so they try to complete themselves by robbing neighbouring molecules. This can set up a chain reaction of damage until the free radical is disarmed by an anti-oxidant, for example, vitamin C. Free radicals damage DNA, the code within cells, and the cell wall itself, preventing the proper supply of nutrients into the cell. Free radicals cause aging, cancer and heart disease, as well as weakening the immune system.

We obtain free radicals from many sources. Any combustion process creates free radicals, so car exhaust and factory fumes give us a generous supply. The sun's rays also generate free radicals, which is why people in hot countries are more prone to skin cancer. Heated fats, especially unsaturated fats, generate free radicals. The more unsaturated the oil the more are generated. Anything burnt creates free radicals including toast, smoked or barbecued foods and cigarettes. But free radicals are not completely avoidable. We actually produce them as a result of making energy from 'burning' glucose with oxygen. They can be thought of as our 'nuclear waste' - rather hard to dispose of.

AVOID
- Avoid fried foods as much as possible.
- If you do fry, use olive oil or butter, never polyunsaturated oils.
- Avoid excessive exposure to strong sunlight.
- Minimise your consumption of smoked or barbecued foods.
- Avoid smoking and smoky atmospheres.
- Don't live in a polluted area.
- Don't eat rancid nuts or seeds.

PROTECT
- Supplement your diet with the anti-oxidant nutrients, vitamins A, C and E, selenium and zinc.
- Exercise at least twice a week.
- Practice relaxation or meditation techniques involving methods for deepening your breathing. This helps bring oxygen to your cells and combat the effects of free radicals.

How To Detoxify Yourself
Most of our detoxifying systems are already partially overloaded so it is important to have times in the year where you give your body a chance to detoxify itself. The first place to start is the digestive tract. Toxins accumulate in the digestive tract, and for a number of reasons we may lose the balance between beneficial bacteria and unwanted micro-organisms such as candida albicans. These produce even

more toxins, while beneficial bacteria actually help to detoxify some pollutants.

Having cleansed your system the next step is to allow your body to detoxify old, stored up toxins. This is speeded up by giving the body short breaks from dealing with current toxic substances in your diet. I recommend having either just fresh fruit and mineral water, or just water for one day a week for six weeks.

There are basically three ways the body detoxifies and stays free of toxins, which it will naturally do when given the chance. The first is competition. Many pollutants compete with nutrient for both absorption and incorporation into cells, once inside the body. By providing those competitive nutrients the body is protected. The minerals calcium and zinc are most important, with magnesium and selenium having a small role to play with some specific pollutants. These pollutants now have to be removed from the body which is helped by the presence of 'chelating' compounds which latch onto and remove these undesirables. Vitamin C is the most important natural chelator.

But not all toxins are removed in this way. Perhaps the majority, including pesticides, some food additives, free radicals and naturally occurring harmful substances in food go through a special detoxification carried out be enzymes in the liver, the purpose of which is to change their form into something that is either non-toxic or can be excreted from the body. Most pesticides, for example, cannot be eliminated from the body without this transformation. The process is called biotransformation. This process actually gives rise to the formation of more free radicals which can then be disarmed by anti-oxidant nutrients primarily vitamin A, C, E, selenium and zinc. All these nutrients concentrate in the liver for this very purpose. Supplementing extra anti-oxidants helps speed up detoxification.

Once your system is detoxified, and you've reduced your overall intake of pollution, you now have the means to stay one step ahead in our unhealthy environment and protect yourself from pollution.

10
PROMOTING BEAUTY FROM THE INSIDE

Y our skin is a mirror for your diet. Although some people appear to have good skin whatever they eat, ultimately you cannot maintain good skin and a youthful body without good nutrition. Good nutrition helps slow down the ageing process, maintains skin suppleness, and tone and decreases spots. Beauty comes from the inside.

The skin does many things for us. It is our first line of defence against bacteria and viruses. We also eliminate unwanted substances through the skin, including toxic metals and body acids, plus a litre of water a day. Most of all, the skin keeps our insides in, in other words makes us a container of all the different chemicals from which we are made, the most important being water. We are, after all, sixty five per cent water.

The skin itself is made out of skin cells. These cells die off as they come to the surface. So the surface of our face is actually dead cells. Within a month you effectively replace your entire skin with new cells. The health of these new cells helps to determine the health of your skin.

Think Zinc

These new cells are made according to your special code, or blueprint, laid down in the DNA molecule, found within all cells. When a new cell is formed it is built according to your blueprint - that is, if you have enough nutrients, especially zinc, in your diet. The body is dependent of vitamins and minerals in order to put together the different proteins that make up a new skin cell. Also, when cells get damaged the body is once more dependent on these nutrients to effect repair. The most important nutrients are zinc, selenium, vitamin C and E plus the B Complex, especially vitamin B6. While these nutrients are important for healthy skin, they're doubly important if you want to heal your skin, for example repair scar tissue that naturally develops after spots.

Anti-Oxidants - The Skin Protectors

One of the reasons skin loses its elasticity is because the elastic bonds become bound up due to damage caused by free radicals. This is why excessive exposure to the sun causes loss of skin elasticity even if the skin is well moisturised. This 'oxidation' occurs all around us. When you leave the lid off an oil based paint the paint becomes hard. When you continually heat up oil, on cooling it becomes solid. The same thing is happening to your skin and face every day.

Fortunately, the body is equipped with anti-oxidants. Vitamins A, C and E are powerful anti-oxidants and help to protect the face from this ageing process. Vitamin E helps to heal the skin and can be applied externally as well as taken in through diet and supplements. Vitamin C is one of the most important nutrients of all. Collagen, the 'glue' between cells, cannot be made without vitamin C. With mild vitamin C deficiency the skin literally droops. With severe deficiency the skin starts to break down, hence the bleeding gums that indicate scurvy, severe vitamin C deficiency. Ideal intakes of vitamin C are between 1 and 5 grams a day. Vitamin C protects us from so many unavoidable hazards of twentieth century living. Pollution, smoke, the effects of alcohol, viruses and the free radicals that are responsible for the ageing of all cells.

A Carrot A Day

Vitamin A plays a special role in the care of the skin and face. As well as protecting the skin from free radicals it is absolutely vital for the production of the outside layer of the skin. If not enough vitamin A reaches your skin it may become rough and flaky. Vitamin A also helps to regulate the oil balance, hence both dry and oily skin can be a sign of insufficient vitamin A levels. According to Doctors Passwater and Cranton, who have researched the effects of nutrients on the body "the most important factor may be the role zinc plays in transporting vitamin A to the skin. Vitamin A is vital to skin health." Nowadays many people are low in zinc, and hence suffer from the apparent effects of not enough vitamin A.

There are two forms of vitamin A: one from vegetable sources, known as beta-carotene; and the other from animal sources, known as retinol. Beta-carotene has to be converted into retinol before it can be used and, once you have enough retinol, very little is converted. Hence it is not toxic even in very large amounts. Retinol, the animal form, is toxic at high levels and occasionally there are reports of toxicity resulting from excessive intake. For example, a woman in the US developed toxicity from eating liver three times a day and taking supplements. It turned out also that the animal feed had also been heavily enriched with vitamin A! But, provided you don't eat liver three times a day you can safely take in up to 10,000 ius of retinol, and as much beta-carotene as you like without risk.

Beta-carotene is rich in carrots and other red, orange or yellow fruits and vegetables. It is rich in beetroot, watermelon, apricots and tomatoes. These are excellent foods for the skin. A carrot a day is a good way of ensuring an adequate intake of beta-carotene.

The Fats of Life

Not all fats are bad for you. Essential fatty acids, founds in fish, nuts, seeds and their oil, are essential for life itself - and for healthy skin. These essential fatty acids form part of the cell's very structure, and are also used to make hormone like substances in the body called prostaglandins.

Prostaglandins do many things. They regulate the release of sebum, oil which protects the skin, although in excess it contributes to blocked pores. They also control all inflammatory reactions. Eczema, dermatitis, psoriasis and allergies involve inflammation that may be helped by the proper supply of essential fatty acids.[1] Prostaglandins also keep the immune system strong. Once more, zinc is critical for the conversion of essential fatty acids to prostaglandins. So is vitamin B6 and magnesium. On the other hand, stress, alcohol, smoking and saturated fat all block the conversion. Another way of ensuring a good prostaglandin activity is to take in a fatty acid called gamma linolenic acid, which is half-way converted to prostaglandins. Gamma linolenic acid, or GLA for short, occurs naturally in evening primrose oil, borage oil and blackcurrant seed oil.

Feeding the Skin

Of course, there's no point taking in a good supply of vitamins, minerals and essential fatty acids if you're diet is awful. We all need a good intake of complex carbohydrates (that's wholegrains, lentils, beans, rice, vegetables); protein from non-fatty sources such as fish, free-range chicken, eggs, a little dairy produce, beans, lentils, nuts and seeds; plus some essential fatty acids from nuts and seeds. Fruit is also excellent because the natural fruit sugar releases slowly giving us energy, apart from the many vitamins, including vitamin C, found in fruit.

Sugar and refined carbohydrates (white bread, biscuits, cakes etc.) are devoid of nutrients and encourage infection in the skin. The unwanted bacteria in the skin feed off sugar. Too much fat from meat, cheese, butter and other spreads and high fat junk foods block the pores of the skin and encourages rapid ageing. Cigarettes destroy nutrients at an alarming rate, as does alcohol, which also dehydrates the body. Coffee and tea have the same effect.

So, for a healthy skin and young face: avoid high fat and fried foods; avoid sugar and foods containing sugar; eat plenty of fruit and fresh vegetables; drink at least one pint of water and/or diluted fruit juices and herb teas, daily; reduce your intake of dairy products; ensure an adequate intake of essential fatty acids, either from nuts, seeds or salad dressings made with cold-pressed sesame or sunflower oil; reduce or avoid coffee, strong tea, cigarettes and alcohol. In other words, pursue optimum nutrition.

11

BREAKING THE FAT BARRIER

The conventional approach to weight loss says this: calories in (from food) less calories out (from exercise) ends up as a wadge around your middle. Of course, there is truth in this simple equation. But is this all there is to weight loss? Consider these questions. Why are some people obese even though they eat very little? Why can some people eat like a horse and never get fat? Why do dieters often put on weight after dieting? Should we be dieting all the time?

If the calorie equation was as simple as many suggest then, since one pound of body fat is roughly equivalent to 4,000 calories, eating 40,000 calories less each year would mean losing 10lb in the first year, and 7 stone by the tenth year. All by eating one less apple a day, because an apple provides 100 calories or 36,500 a year. The calorie equation for exercise is equally ridiculous. Cycle vigourously for 15 minutes each day and you will lose 10lb in the first year - quite possibly, but 7 stone after ten years? No chance. However, according to calorie theory, one apple a day undoes all that hard work.

How Fat Burning Works

The missing link in the equation is your metabolism: how efficient your body is at turning food into energy. In other words it isn't just about the quantity of food, but the quality of the food you eat, and how well your body can handle it. Modern approaches to weight loss focus on helping the body to burn fat by encouraging proper metabolism, as well as restricting overeating.

The fat-burning approach to weight loss, first proposed in my book, the Metabolic Diet, is a proven method of painless weight control resulting in a consistent weight loss of over one pound a week. In a study in Northern Ireland this approach was compared to Unislim, a system similar to Weightwatchers including regular meetings to help motivate participants. After twelve weeks the fat burners had lost, on average, 14 pounds compared to 2 pounds on the Unislim programme. Four magazines put this approach to the test. This is what they concluded:

The Diet proved such a success with readers, that they decided to put three people on the diet for three months and watch what happened. Ian went from 15 stone 5lbs to 14 stone and felt so good that he gave up smoking. Sabine wanted to lose at least 7 lbs and lost 10 lbs. Her only problem was coping with the extra energy. Gina lost 10 lbs and continues to lose 1-2 lbs a week. All felt positively healthy on the diet. **Woman's Realm Magazine.**

"After the first few days I began to feel wonderful - alert and fit and thoroughly detoxified, with no more puffy eyes staring back from the bathroom mirror. There's no shortage of recipe ideas. I lost 10 lbs in a month and regained 2 lbs on holiday, but will soon whittle that off by eating sensibly." **Sunday Times Magazine.**

"Weight loss: 4 lbs to 7 lbs in four weeks. Verdict: Makes you look and feel good. Side effects: None." **Time Out Magazine.**

"Increased alertness was a significant benefit. By the third day, everybody felt well - alert on rising, and three of us (including me) were bounding about full of the joys of spring. Two out of ten felt hungry, but the rest said that, as far as hunger was concerned, it was a comparatively easy diet to stick to. Mrs Kilby noted by day four that her concentration had improved, and this was backed up by comments from other testers. Nobody had that weak and wobbly feeling associated with dieting. By the end of the week, everybody had stayed the course. Weight loss over the week varied from 3 lbs to 7 lbs, 4-5 lbs being the average." **She Magazine.**

Numerous personal letters have confirmed these findings. Britain's first 'fatburner' said this: "I lost three stone. I have never felt hungry on this diet. I know I'll never go back to eating like I used to." Perhaps most significant is the finding that the vast majority of these people have maintained their reduced weight. So how does this approach work? Fatburning is based on three key principles: balancing you diet both for quality and quantity; improving your metabolism; and the right kind of exercise.

Balancing Your Diet

Balancing your diet from the point of view of weight loss means much more than eating less fat. In fact, in the quest to eliminate calories by avoiding fat many diets are deficient in essential fatty acids which are vital to the body's metabolism. So, although fat intake should be low diets should contain sources of essential fatty acids, found in nuts, seeds and their oils.

Since a pound of fat has almost double the calories of a pound of carbohydrate a high carbohydrate diet is essential. However, the kind of carbohydrate is vital. Slow releasing carbohydrates, as found in beans, lentils, unprocessed whole grains such as brown rice, and fruit, help to keep the blood sugar level even. Since we get hungry when our blood sugar level drops, but, when our blood sugar level is too high, we turn the excess into fat, keeping the blood sugar level balanced is critical to weight control.

Fibre is an important constituent of your diet. As well as keeping the digestive system healthy it helps the 'slow-release' of carbohydrates into the body and gives a sensation of fullness, thereby decreasing appetite. Our knowledge of fibre and the best sources of fibre has been completely revised in the last five years. We now know that there are important fibres in fruit, vegetables, beans and lentils, as well as whole grains. Some of the fibres in vegetables are increasingly destroyed with cooking, so raw food is recommended. Some fibres are made out of protein, while the old definition of fibre was 'indigestible carbohydrate'. With the right diet there is simply no need to add extra fibre.

Improving Your Metabolism

Metabolism is the process of turning food into energy (catabolism) or using it for building materials (anabolism). In order to slim you want to turn food into energy, rather than fat; burn off unwanted fat; and increase lean muscle to improve your fitness and body shape. In order to achieve this you need to do two things: Give the body the right fuel; and 'tune-up' your metabolism. While a car will run further on the right fuel, it will run faster and further when the engine is tuned up.

The best fuel for the body is slow-releasing carbohydrates, either complex carbohydrates found in lentils, beans, vegetables and unprocessed whole grains, or simple carbohydrates found in most fruit. (Although fruit contains a simple sugar, fructose, this cannot be used directly by the body and first has to be converted into glucose. It is this delay that classifies most fruit as 'slow releasing'. Grapes and dates are exceptions.) These foods help to keep the blood sugar level even.

Stress and stimulants have a profound effect on blood sugar by stimulating the release of emergency stores of sugar in the body. For this reason stimulants such as tea, coffee, chocolate and cigarettes are best avoided or reduced. In the short term these substances may appear to help you keep an even weight, but in the long-term their effect is opposite. Almost all dieters as well as 'stimulant addicts' have an underlying blood sugar imbalance. If a smoker stops smoking but does not correct the underlying blood sugar imbalance they're likely to crave another stimulant like sugar or coffee. The underlying blood sugar imbalance must be put right to correct obesity in the long-run. As well as eating complex carbohydrates and cutting down on stimulants, specific vitamins and minerals have an important part to play.

No less than 13 vitamins and minerals are needed to turn glucose into energy. Having adequate supplies of these is critical for proper metabolism. This is what the most important ones do:

B3 (niacin) is one of the constituents of GTF (glucose tolerance factor) which again helps to keep blood sugar levels even. 100mg a day is recommended.

B6 is fundamental for the production of enzymes, which ensure smooth digestion. It is also required for the production of sex hormones and insulin, helping to keep blood sugar levels stable. 100mg a day of B6 is recommended.

Vitamin C has many roles to play in weight control. Most of all it is needed in proper hormone production and is involved in the conversion of glucose to energy in the cell. 1 to 3g per day is recommended.

Chromium is the major nutrient in GTF released every time our blood sugar level rises. GTF makes insulin more effective and is crucial for proper blood sugar balance. 100mcg per day is recommended.

Zinc is probably the most deficient nutrient in Britain. It is involved in some 200 enzyme reactions, including the energy cycle. Deficiency causes abnormal appetite control and disperceptions about body size. 15mg a day is recommended.

These nutrients need to be supplemented every day, together with a good, all-round multivitamin and mineral supplement.

Air-obics

The two most important nutrients, air and water, are often overlooked. Metabolism depends on a good supply of oxygen. Without enough oxygen metabolism is very sluggish. The right kind of exercise, known as aerobic exercise, stimulates breathing to take in enough oxygen to allow exercising muscles to perform. If the exercise is too severe, for example sprinting, muscle cells cannot take in enough oxygen. The best kinds of exercise should raise your heartbeat to 80% of your maximum heart rate (which is 200 beats per minute less your age) and keep it there for at least 12 minutes. So jogging, cycling, swimming, brisk walking, and aerobics classes are all good.

Aerobic exercise has many benefits. It strengthens your heart, oxygenates body tissues, keeps you fit and in shape, but most of all, it boosts your metabolism. During vigorous exercise your rate of metabolism can increase ten-fold, but even after 48 hours after exercise your metabolic rate may still be increased. Studies have shown that the metabolic rate of exercisers is still 25% higher 15 hours after exercise. Exercising as little as three times a week for twenty minutes is likely to make a substantial difference in the long-term.

These three principles, when incorporated into your life, are virtually guaranteed to produce results. The principles in Part Three of this book will help to get you started. Optimum nutrition is, after all, the key to balancing your metabolism and maintaining the right weight.

12
CONQUERING EATING DISORDERS

For many people, especially teenagers, gaining weight is not the problem, it's losing it. Eating disorders including anorexia nervosa and bulimia, in which the sufferer may binge and then make themselves sick, effect thousands of people and are very much on the increase.

One of the greatest shortcomings of human logic is the unquestioned belief that psychological problems, be it of behaviour or intelligence, are influenced only by psychological factors, and that physiological problems are influenced only by physiological factors. This presupposes that mind and body are separate, that the energy of mind and of body are two different things. Our experience contradicts this. Alcohol alters your state of mind. Psychological stress makes muscles tense. Ask a chemist, an anatomist and a psychologist to define where the mind starts and the body ends and they will find that the two are intimately interconnected. The same is especially true of anorexia because it is a behavioural disorder involving eating, a physiological event.

Anorexia was first identified by Dr. William Gull in 1874. He advocated "The patient should be fed at regular intervals, and surrounded by persons who could have moral control over them, relations and friends being generally the worst attendants." Today, treatment is often essentially the same, summed up as 'drug them, feed them and let them get on with their lives' in an article in the

Guardian describing treatment in 'leading hospitals'. The 'modern' approach includes 'behaviour therapy' i.e. rewards and privileges, and drugs to induce compliance. The drugs include psychotropic drugs such as chlorpromazine, sedatives and anti-depressants. The diet is high carbohydrate, sometimes as much as 5,000 kcals, with little regard to quality.

The idea that nutrition, or malnutrition could play in the development and treatment of this condition did not really emerge until the 1980s when scientists began to realise just how similar the symptoms and risk factors of anorexia and zinc deficiency were. As early as 1973 two zinc researchers, Hambidge and Silverman, concluded that, "whenever there is appetite loss in children zinc deficiency should be suspected".[1] In 1979, Bakan, a Canadian health researcher noticed that the symptoms of anorexia and zinc deficiency were similar in a number of respects and proposed that clinical trials be undertaken to test its effectiveness in treatment.[2] Meanwhile, David Horrobin, most renowned for his research into evening primrose oil, proposed that "anorexia nervosa is due to a combined deficiency of zinc and EFA's."[3]

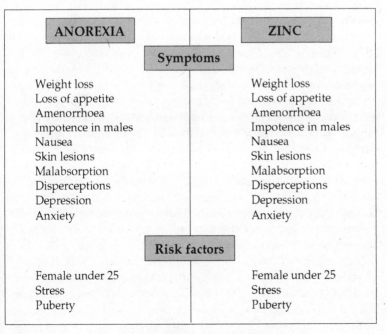

ANOREXIA	ZINC
Symptoms	
Weight loss	Weight loss
Loss of appetite	Loss of appetite
Amenorrhoea	Amenorrhoea
Impotence in males	Impotence in males
Nausea	Nausea
Skin lesions	Skin lesions
Malabsorption	Malabsorption
Disperceptions	Disperceptions
Depression	Depression
Anxiety	Anxiety
Risk factors	
Female under 25	Female under 25
Stress	Stress
Puberty	Puberty

Figure 9   *Symptoms of Anorexia Compared to Zinc Deficiency*

Zinc Hypothesis Confirmed

In 1980 the first trial started at the University of Kentucky. The researchers discovered that 10 out 13 patients admitted with anorexia and 8 out of 14 patients with bulimia were zinc deficient on admission. After vigourous refeeding they became even more zinc deficient.[4] Since zinc is required to digest and utilise protein, from which body tissue is made, they recommended that extra zinc, above that required to correct deficiency, should be given as the anorexic starts to eat and gain weight.

In 1984 the penny dropped with two important research findings and the first case of an anorexic treated with zinc. The first study showed that animals deprived of zinc very rapidly developed loss of appetite, and that if these animals were force fed a zinc deficient diet to gain weight they became seriously ill.[5] The second study showed that zinc deficiency damages the intestinal wall and therefore the absorption of nutrients, including zinc, potentially leading to a vicious spiral of deficiency.[6]

Then, in 1984 Professor Bryce-Smith, renowned for his exposure of the dangers of lead, and Dr.Simpson, a doctor from Reading, reported the first case of anorexia treated with zinc. The patient was a thirteen year-old girl, tearful and depressed, weighing 37kg. She was referred to a consultant psychiatrist, but, despite counselling, three months later her weight was 31.5 kg (under 5 stone). Within two months of zinc supplementation at a level of 45mg per day her weight returned to 44.5kg, she was cheerful again, and tests for zinc deficiency were normal.[7]

Scientists all over the world started to test the effects of zinc on anorexia. Two Swedish doctors at the University of Goteburg reported that "our initial patient is currently maintained on zinc supplementation (45mg per day). She is doing very well: her weight as well as her menstruations are normalised."[8] Meanwhile, the first double-blind trial with 15 anorexics was being carried out at the University of California. The 1987 the researchers reported their findings... "Zinc supplementation was followed by a decrease in depression and anxiety. Our data suggest that individuals with anorexia nervosa may be at risk for zinc deficiency and may respond favourably after zinc supplementation."[9] By 1990 many researchers had found that over 50 per cent of anorexic patients showed clear biochemical evidence of zinc deficiency.[10]

Mind or Body?

The fact that high levels of zinc supplementation help to treat anorexia does not mean the cause of anorexia is zinc deficiency. Psychological issues may, and probably do, bring about change in the eating habits of susceptible people. By avoiding eating a young girl can repress the signs of growing up. Menstruation stops, breast size decreases and the body stays small. Starvation induces a kind of 'high' by stimulating changes in important brain chemicals, that may help to block out difficult feelings and issues that are too hard to face. But once the route of not eating is chosen and becomes established zinc deficiency is almost inevitable due to both poor intake and poor absorption. With it comes a further loss of appetite and even more depression, disperceptions, and the inability to cope with the stresses that face many adolescents, especially girls, growing up in the 1990s.

The optimum nutrition approach to help someone with anorexia, or bulimia, is best carried out alongside work with a skilled psychotherapist. The nutritional approach emphasizes quality of food rather than quantity, including supplements to ensure vitamin and mineral sufficiency, and of course 45mg of elemental zinc per day, halving the level once weight gain is achieved and maintained.

13
BALANCING SEX HORMONES AND FEMALE HEALTH

Hormones are chemical messengers which control vital processes throughout the body. For example, hormones control our rate of metabolism, the level of glucose in the blood, the balance of calcium, our response to stress and the sexual cycle. Different phases of our life are marked by hormonal changes. These periods of transition often make extra demands on our nutritional needs. For this reason symptoms of nutrient deficiency often appear at puberty, during pregnancy or at the menopause. For women, symptoms may become more pronounced prior to menstruation. The greatest nutritional imbalances result is a loss of fertility in both male and female.

Maximising Fertility

One in every four couples suffers from some degree of infertility. For some, this means having fewer children than they want; for most, it means no children at all. And for couples who are fertile getting pregnant is not the easy matter that it is commonly thought to be. The average length of time taken to get pregnant is six months, although 18 months is not uncommon. Unless fertility tests show otherwise, failure to conceive within 18 months does not necessarily mean that you are completely infertile.

Fertility and the speed of conception depend on many factors, some psychological, some physical and some nutritional.

Conceptions are very high during holiday periods, for example, since stress - a major factor in infertility - is reduced. Knowing how to time intercourse to coincide with ovulation (the release of the female egg to be fertilised by the sperm) greatly increases the chances of conception. Also, your nutrition and especially your vitamin status play a crucial role.

Vitamins for Fertility

The male is responsible in about a third of infertility cases. It should be stressed that infertility has nothing to do with sexual virility, which is usually not affected. The usual test for infertility in a man involves a sperm count - the higher the sperm count, the greater the fertility. A recent study has shown that extra vitamin C increased sperm count as well as sperm mobility, but exactly why this is so is not yet known. Likewise, vitamin E deficiency has been found to induce sterility in both sexes by causing damage to the reproductive tissues. Unfortunately, however, simply taking vitamin E will not reverse the condition if you are sterile.

The high rate of infertility among diabetics may provide us with a clue. Diabetics are frequently low in vitamin A, which is essential for making the male sex hormones. Vitamin A is dependent on zinc to be released from the liver. Of all the nutrients known to affect male fertility, zinc is perhaps the best researched. Signs of zinc deficiency include late sexual maturation, small sex organs and infertility. With adequate supplements of zinc these problems can be corrected. Dr Carl Pfeiffer also found a high degree of impotence and infertility in male patients who suffer from zinc deficiency. 'With adequate dosage of vitamin B6 and zinc,' he wrote, 'the sexual ability of the male should return in one or two months' time.'[1] In view of the fact that the average dietary intake of zinc has been found to be substantially lower at 7.9mg than the intake of 15mg recommended by the National Research Council, the effects of zinc on fertility may be quite substantial and widespread. Zinc is found in high concentrations in the sex glands of the male and also in the sperm itself. There it is needed to make the outer layer and the tail and is therefore essential for healthy sperm. As much as 1.4mg of zinc is lost with each ejaculation, so a prolific sex life and an inadequate diet would put you at risk! In the nineteenth century many patients were diagnosed as having 'masturbation insanity' - perhaps the earliest suggestion of a link between zinc, sex and mental illness. There may be more than an element of truth in the old saying that masturbation makes you blind and stunts your growth, since both of these are signs of zinc deficiency!

For women, zinc is also crucial. Problems of fertility, sex drive and menstruation have all been linked to inadequate levels of zinc. The sex hormone, gonadotrophin, needs zinc and vitamin B6 to be produced in adequate quantities. Vitamin B6 together with zinc beneficially affect every part of the female sexual cycle. They increase desire for sex, alleviate premenstrual problems, ease sickness in pregnancy and post-natal depression, and increase the chances of a healthy baby.

Contraception: Pros and Cons

It is not just dietary deficiency that can cause problems with zinc and vitamin B6, but also the birth control pill. The link was discovered when 80mg of B6 helped those suffering from depression induced by the pill. The pill also induces deficiencies in vitamin C and the B vitamins, especially B12.[2] Since the pill also elevates the level of copper, which has been associated with increased birth defects, one might end up taking vitamin and mineral pills to counteract the effects of this contraceptive! A much better alternative is to switch to a safer form of birth control: since the use of the pill has been associated with migraine headaches, cervical cancer and an increase in depression and suicide among young women. Medical researcher Ellen Grant says, 'Women have been sacrificed to the god of perfect contraception', and advises strongly against the pill. Unfortunately, its effects do not stop when you cease taking it; the chance of having an abnormal baby has already been increased from 0.9 to 4.3 per cent. Also, a greater incidence of allergies is now being discovered among children of mothers who used to take the pill. Not surprisingly, fertility is also affected. So what are the alternatives?

The coil or IUD (intra-uterine device) may not be ideal. Many types of coil are made from copper and these may elevate levels of this potentially toxic metal in the body. Since copper is a strong enemy of zinc, zinc deficiency could be increased. Copper is both an essential and toxic mineral frequently high in drinking water. So, if your water is high in copper any potential sources of extra copper are best avoided. Non-copper IUDs do not present this problem.

Natural Methods of Birth Control

Unlike the pill or coil, natural methods of birth control do not interfere with the cycle of ovulation (the release of the egg from the ovary) and menstruation (the discharge of the nourishing part of the uterus in which a fertilised egg would implant). During this cycle, which can vary from 23 to 35 days, there is only one day in which the egg is available for fertilisation. This is the point of ovulation. However, sperm usually live for three days; under excellent conditions, they can survive for five days (a longer survival rate is extremely rare). If one knew exactly when ovulation occurred, abstinence from sex for five days (or the use of a diaphragm or condom) would reduce the chance of pregnancy, while frequent sex during this time would dramatically increase it. How, then, do you find out when ovulation occurs?

The ways to find out can be briefly summarised in three groups. Perhaps the best known is the rhythm method, which predicts ovulation a certain number of days after menstruation every month, but this is not a method to be recommended to those whose cycle is not absolutely regular. The temperature method depends on taking the body temperature at different times of the month, since it rises after ovulation due to an increase in the hormone progesterone. The disadvantage of this method is that it can only tell you after ovulation has occurred: it cannot predict it in advance.

A third method is expounded by Dr E Billings in her book, The Billings Method (Allen Lane, 1981). It is based on the discovery that a different type of vaginal mucus is produced just before ovulation. If you can learn to recognise this accurately, you will know just when to avoid intercourse if you do not want to become pregnant and, of course, just when you are most fertile if you are trying for a child. Most researchers report a success rate of 97 to 99 per cent using this method of birth control, provided that intercourse is abstained from for just a few days in each cycle.

Vitamins for a Healthy Pregnancy

Optimum nutrition can greatly improve your chances of having a healthy pregnancy. Even the slightest deficiencies during pregnancy can have serious effects on the health of the offspring, and the idea that birth defects are often caused by nutritional imbalances in the mother is rapidly gaining wider acceptance. So far, slight deficiencies of vitamin B1, B2, B6, folic acid, zinc, iron, calcium and magnesium have all been linked to birth abnormalities.[3] So too have excesses of toxic metals, especially lead, cadmium and copper.[4] Severe deficiencies of any vitamin will cause birth abnormalities, since a vitamin by definition is necessary for maintaining normal growth.

Naturally, a healthy pregnancy will depend on a greater supply than normal of all these nutrients since the needs of a growing foetus, together with her own needs, put extra demands on the expectant mother.

Spina bifida, a condition in which the neural tube doesn't develop properly, has been strongly linked to a lack of folic acid in the mother's diet and probably of other nutrients too.[5] A survey of 23,000 women found that those who supplemented their diet with a multivitamin including folic acid during the first six weeks of pregnancy had a 75% lower incidence of neural tube defects than those who didn't.[6] The incidence of this condition is far higher where mothers have had a nutritionally poor diet for the first three months of pregnancy. One study found that dietary counselling alone did lower the rate of spina bifida in those mothers at risk, but that the administration of extra folic acid, on its own or in a multivitamin preparation, resulted in a much lower number of babies with neural tube defects. Since the recommended folic acid intake is 300mcg per day and the average intake is between 109 and 203mcg per day, a supplement of 200mcg per day is recommended for those intending to become pregnant.

During the first three months of pregnancy all the organs of the body are completely formed. It is during this period - and, of course, before - that optimum nutrition is most important. Yet many women experience continual sickness and don't feel like eating healthily. Misnamed 'morning' sickness, this condition has been accepted as normal during the first three months of pregnancy. Probably due to increases in a hormone called HCG, women with poor diets are particularly at risk. During pregnancy the need for vitamin B6, B12, folic acid, iron and zinc all increase; extra supplements of these usually stop even the worst cases of pregnancy sickness. Eating small, frequent amounts of fruit or complex carbohydrates like nuts, seeds or wholegrains often helps. However, the best approach is to ensure optimum nutrition well before pregnancy. We followed up four women on optimum programmes before and during pregnancy - the average number of days in which nausea or sickness was reported was two days. Yet for some women nausea continues throughout the entire pregnancy!

Another common complication of pregnancy is called pre-eclamptic toxaemia, consisting of an increase in blood pressure, oedema (swelling) and an excess level of protein in the urine. Many theories abound as to why this occurs, but once more optimum nutrition is a vital factor. One of my clients who had had pre-eclamptic toxaemia during her previous pregnancy improved her diet and added nutritional supplements: her second pregnancy was entirely healthy and she didn't even experience nausea.

For the mother, optimum nutrition before and during pregnancy ensures a healthier pregnancy with fewer complications, resulting in a healthier and heavier baby. Your supplement programme should include 200 mcg of folic acid, 20mcg of vitamin B12, 200mg of Vitamin B6, 15mg of zinc, 500mg of calcium, 250mg of magnesium and 12mg of iron. Do not take more than 10,000iu of vitamin A, and have a hair mineral analysis to check for excesses of copper, lead or cadmium. My book, The Better Pregnancy Diet (ION Press), goes into this subject in much more detail, covering all important issues from pre-conception up to age 5 of the child.

PMT - the Curse that can be Cured

Premenstrual problems were, until relatively recently, accepted as a woman's lot. Yet these symptoms - which include depression, tension, headaches, breast tenderness, bloating, low energy and irritability - are in most cases avoidable. Classically, they occur in the week preceding menstruation, though a small percentage of women have the symptoms from the middle of the cycle, coinciding with ovulation. Since premenstrual problems are a result of hormonal changes, hormone treatment has been used to correct them. But the use of such drug treatment must be seriously questioned as it does disrupt the body's chemistry and has been associated with a greater risk of cancer. The effectiveness of vitamin B6 has now been shown in some studies to help 70 per cent of premenstrual sufferers.[7] More recently, research has focused on the role of GLA (gamma linolenic acid), an essential fatty acid found in the oil of the evening primrose.[8] GLA's high success rate of 60 per cent is almost certainly due to its role in making prostaglandins, which are hormone-like substances in the body. Vitamin B6, zinc and magnesium are all required to make prostaglandins and, perhaps for this reason, have been shown to help PMT sufferers.[9] But why are so many women deficient in these nutrients?

We selected a group of women with serious premenstrual problems and, rather than use a single nutrient like B6 or GLA, calculated their optimum nutritional requirements. After all, since nutrients work together in the body and should be supplied together in the diet, to treat a condition with one nutrient alone is against all the principles of optimum nutrition.

Out of nine women we asked an independent doctor to select those with the most pronounced premenstrual problems. We then gave them the appropriate vitamin and mineral supplements. Each participant then recorded her tiredness, depression, bloatedness, tension and headaches over the next four menstrual cycles.

The results clearly indicated that there was a substantial improvement for each premenstrual health problem of between 55 and 85 per cent. Expressed as an average, a person on such a programme could expect a 66 per cent improvement in each of these premenstrual problems within three months. The testimonials overleaf illustrate the results experienced by many women who have tried the nutritional approach to menstrual problems.

Optimum Nutrition and the Menopause

The menopause is a natural transition from the child-bearing phase of life for a woman. It occurs most often between ages 45 and 50, sometimes without any unpleasant symptoms, and sometimes with a whole host of symptoms, the most common being hot flushes, night sweats, tiredness, headaches, irritability, depression and joint pains. These may occur for just a few months up to 18 months.

There is increasing evidence that optimum nutrition can alleviate many of these symptoms and shorten their duration. Factors that have been shown to help are correcting underlying blood sugar imbalances or allergies, and supplementation with vitamin E[10], B complex, calcium, magnesium and zinc. Essential fatty acids such as evening primrose oil may also be of help. One study at ION found the addition of vitamin E to relieve symptoms.[11] A later trial found even better results using a combination of calcium, magnesium, vitamin D and E.[12] In this study there was a 62.7% reduction in reported symptoms in a group of nineteen women over a 12 week period. While improved diet may help, diet plus supplements seems to be most effective.[13]

With optimum nutrition there is no doubt that all aspects of life to do with the sexual cycle and fertility can be improved.

SUBJECT 1

BEFORE Doctor's report 'She has had erratic periods since the age of 12. In 1978 she started progesterone therapy to relieve her premenstrual irrational outbursts, depression, lethargy and bloatedness. It helped, but she still experienced depression, weepiness, bloatedness and irrational behaviour up to five days before her period.'

Subject's report 'Five days before my period I can't get up in the morning and my muscles feel weak. I put on weight, my eyes go puffy and I feel bloated. I also get very irritable and tense, and have difficulty sleeping. I always get headaches.'

AFTER Doctor's report 'Improved considerably for one month, then relapsed, now improving again. More energy, headaches gone completely, sleep improved, less irritable.'

Subject's report 'Getting up is no longer a problem, I have much more energy. My bloatedness is better, depression is better, I'm much less irritable, I've had no headaches and sleep is no problem. I've noticed all symptoms occur later. In fact, my period is due in two days and I have no symptoms at all.'

SUBJECT 2

BEFORE Doctor's report 'Smokes 40 a day; coughs. Irregular periods before going on the pill in 1979. Symptoms of tension, nervousness, tearfulness, depression and lack of energy, not exclusively before period.'

Subject's report 'I begin to feel bloated and heavy two days before my period. I get depressed, tearful and am very easily upset. I feel tense and my skin condition gets worse and I get more spots.'

AFTER Doctor's report 'Significant improvement in all symptoms. Has not been warned of periods prior to their onset during this time.'

Subject's report 'Haven't noticed bloatedness at all. Indigestion and wind are much better. I don't get the tension, depression and tears before my period. My skin is much better, it isn't dry and flaky like before, I have no dandruff, my thrush has gone, I've stopped losing hair, my nose is not so blocked, I don't get the prickly sensations in my legs due to my varicose veins, and I no longer get a coated tongue or cracked lips.'

SUBJECT 3

BEFORE Doctor's report 'Previous health history is good. Experiences abdominal pain, depression and irrational emotional outbursts, tension, listlessness and some weight gain prior to period. Also sometimes headaches.'

Subject's report 'I experience tiredness and lethargy, both in body and mind, usually one day before period. I get bloated, depressed and tense four days before, and occasionally get a headache on the side of my head when waking.'

AFTER Doctor's report 'Improvement in energy, no change in headaches.'

Subject's report 'I've had a definite improvement in energy, both in body and mind. Depression before my period is less noticeable, tension is a little less, there wasn't a lot of bloatedness, and headaches occur at the same time but I get them less frequently. I've noticed my skin is less dry, I've had fewer colds, my cracked lips are better and I haven't had a nose bleed.'

PART 3

YOUR PERSONAL HEALTH PROGRAMME

14

HOW TO WORK OUT YOUR OPTIMUM NUTRITION

How healthy do you want to be? If you want to realise your full potential, mentally and physically, finding out your optimum nutritional requirements is essential. But if your needs are unique, how do you find these out? Since 1980 I have been developing and refining a precise system for analysing people's nutrient needs, based on assessing the major factors that influence the individual's requirements. This system is now used by qualified nutritionists all over the world.

More than 10,000 people have benefitted from this system, so I know what sort of results to expect. They include greater mental alertness, improved memory, more physical energy, better weight control and a reduced risk of degenerative disease. Although many people with diagnosed illnesses have been helped while on a Personal Health Programme, it is not designed to treat illness so much as to prevent it. The claims for 'curing' advanced degenerative diseases with nutrition are often exaggerated. If you suffer from a recognised medical condition, please check that this programme is compatible with any treatment you may already be receiving.

The next two chapters present a simplified version of that system based on questions and answers. It provides a useful assessment of what you need for optimum health and is a good place to start. It does not, however, equate to having a personal assessment of your nutritional needs with a nutrition consultant. This is, of course, highly preferable, and essential for anyone who is currently unwell or suffering from a diagnosed disease. A directory of nutrition consultants qualified to assess your individual needs for optimum health and nutrition is available from the Institute for Optimum Nutrition (ION) 5 Jerdan Place, London SW6 1BE for £1.50.

Factors that Affect Your Nutritional Needs

At least eight factors affect your optimum nutritional requirements. Factors such as your age, sex and amount of exercise are easy to assess. But the effects of pollution, your past health history and, of course, the nutrients (and anti-nutrients) supplied in your diet are not so straightforward to work out. But all these factors and more must be taken into account. There are four basic ways to go about it: diet analysis, biochemical analysis, symptom analysis and lifestyle analysis.

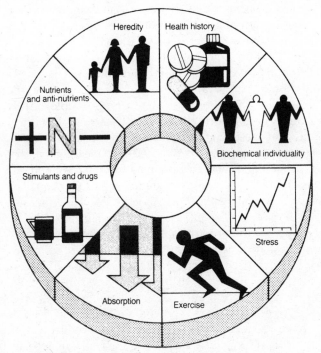

Figure 10 Factors That Effect Nutritional Needs

Diet Analysis

Diet may seem the obvious place to start. By finding out what goes in, one could know what is missing. But unfortunately, a breakdown of foods eaten over, say, a week, cannot take into account the variations in nutrient content in the food, your individual needs, nor how well the nutrient is used when, and if, it is absorbed. I have seen many people who had superficially 'perfect' diets, but still showed signs of vitamin deficiency. For many of these people the problem was poor absorption. These variables make some diet analyses done on a computer less than accurate.

Diet analysis is useful in assessing foods that are known to affect our nutrient needs - such as sugar, salt, coffee, tea, alcohol, food additives and preservatives. Nutrients that make up a large proportion of our food intake, such as fats, carbohydrates, protein and calories, can also be determined reasonably accurate from an analysis of your diet.

Biochemical Analysis

Biochemical tests such as hair mineral analysis or vitamin blood tests give indisputable information about biochemical status and help a nutrition consultant to know the actual nutritional state of your body. But not all of these tests provide useful information to help you build up your nutrition programme.

Any vitamin or mineral test, to be accurate, must reflect the ability of the nutrient to function in the body. For example, iron is a vital constituent of red blood cells; it helps to carry oxygen throughout the body. By measuring the iron status in your cells it is possible to get a good measure of your iron needs. On the other hand, vitamin B6 has no similar direct function to perform in the blood - it is used in other chemical reactions, for example the production of the brain chemical, serotonin, which helps us go to sleep. So a measure of the B6 level in your blood would tell you nothing. In fact, if B6 isn't being used properly in other parts of the body, blood levels may be high, although a state of deficiency exists elsewhere. So for vitamin B6 a clever test has been devised, called a 'functional enzyme test'. Tryptophan, a constituent of protein, is acted upon by enzymes, which turn it into serotonin, a neuro-transmitter in the body. One of these enzymes is dependent on vitamin B6. So if you do not have enough B6, instead of making serotonin you produce a by-product, xanthurenic acid, which is excreted in the urine. By measuring the amount of xanthurenic acid excreted, it is possible to gauge whether you are getting enough B6 and if it is being used properly. This is just one of a number of tests now being used to determine vitamin B6 status.

Because each nutrient has a different function in the body, we cannot say that blood tests are better than urine tests, or that analysis of levels of minerals in the hair provides more accurate information than blood levels. For each nutrient there are different tests depending on what we want to find out. For instance, there are over a dozen tests for zinc deficiency. These involve blood, urine, hair, sweat and even a taste test.

To make an extensive series of tests would be expensive. My number one 'value for money' test is hair mineral analysis, which tells you about mineral status. From a small sample of hair the levels of lead, cadmium, arsenic, aluminium and mercury can be tested: all of these are toxic in excess. Hair mineral analysis also provides useful information about calcium, magnesium, zinc, copper, chromium, selenium and manganese, although these results need careful interpretation.[1] Hair mineral analysis can sometimes pinpoint problems of absorption, reasons for high blood pressure or frequent infections.

To find out vitamin status, I use a series of 'functional enzyme tests', which are more expensive than hair mineral analysis. However, the results of these enzyme tests usually confirm findings already made from deficiency symptom analysis. I mainly use these for 'fine-tuning' or when there is some doubt about the results of a previous test.

Symptom Analysis

Deficiency symptom analysis is the most underestimated method of working out nutritional needs. It is based on over 200 signs and symptoms that have been found in cases of slight vitamin or mineral deficiency. For example, mouth ulcers are associated with vitamin A deficiency, muscle cramps with magnesium deficiency. For many of these symptoms, the mechanism is understood. For example, magnesium is required for muscles to relax. Symptoms such as these can be early warning signs of deficiency. They show us that our bodies are not working perfectly. However, while deficiency in vitamins C, B3 or B5 would all result in reduced energy because they are involved in the production of energy, being low in energy doesn't necessarily mean you're deficient. Perhaps you are just working too hard or not getting enough sleep. However, if you have five different symptoms, all associated with B3 deficiency, then you are much more likely to be needing more vitamin B3 to reach optimum health.

The advantage of deficiency symptom analysis is that health is being measured directly. Results are not dependent on whether you eat oranges that are high in Vitamin C, or whether you absorb and utilise food well, as dietary analysis is. Some people have criticised this method because it relies on subjective information from the person concerned. Yet the large majority of medical diagnoses are in fact based on subjective information from the patient. If you want to find out how someone feels, isn't it obvious to ask? I always ask my clients why they think they're ill. More often than not they're right.

Lifestyle Analysis

These three methods of analysis, diet, symptom and biochemical if properly applied, should define what you need right now to be optimally nourished. But it's good to check that your needs for your particular lifestyle are adequately covered. For example, if you smoke and drink alcohol frequently your nutritional needs will be higher. If you are pregnant, if you live in a city, if you have a high-stress occupation, if you suffer from allergies - all of these factors may alter your needs.

Lifestyle analysis is the fourth piece of the jigsaw puzzle that helps a nutritionist know what you need. The next two chapters tell you how to analyse your diet, your symptoms of deficiency and your lifestyle in order to work out your own Personal Health Programme.

15

YOUR OPTIMUM DIET

B efore foods can give us vitality, hundreds of chemical reactions must take place involving 28 different vitamins and minerals. These micro-nutrients are the real keys that unlock the potential energy in our food.

Your vitality depends upon a careful balance of at least 38 nutrients. They include sources of energy or calories which may come from carbohydrates, fats or proteins; 13 known vitamins, 15 minerals, eight amino acids (which we get when proteins are digested), and two essential fatty acids. Even though the requirement for some minerals, like selenium, is less than a millionth of our requirement for protein, it is no less important. In fact, one third of all chemical reactions in our bodies are dependent on tiny quantities of minerals, and even more on vitamins. Without any one of these nutrients, vitality, energy and ideal weight are just not possible.

Fortunately, deficiency in proteins, fats or carbohydrates is very rare in Europe. Unfortunately, deficiency in vitamins and minerals is not, despite popular belief. Many nutritionists believe that as few as one in ten people receive sufficient vitamins and minerals from their diet for optimum health.

As much as two thirds of the average calorie intake is fat, sugar and refined flours. The calories in sugar are called 'empty' calories because they provide no nutrients. Often hidden in processed foods and snacks, they usually weigh little and instantly satisfy our appetite. For instance, two sweet biscuits provide more calories than a 1lb (0.45kg) of carrots. They are considerably easier to eat, but they provide no vitamins or minerals. If a quarter of your diet by weight, and two thirds by calories, consists of such dismembered foods, there's little room left to get the levels you need of the 38 essential nutrients.

Wheat, for example, has 25 nutrients removed in the refining process that turns it into white flour, yet only four (iron, B1, B2, B3) are replaced. On average, 87 per cent of the vital minerals zinc, chromium and manganese are lost. Have we been short-changed? Processed meats like hamburgers and sausages are no better. The use of inferior meat lowers the nutrient content but increases the calories and saturated fat. Eggs, fish and chicken are nutrient-rich sources of protein, but protein deficiency is rarely a problem.

Vegetables, fruits, nuts and seeds are full of vitality. Tomatoes and lettuce, for example, are packed with vitamins and minerals. The humble potato is also vitality rich (even though an advertising survey found that more people thought ice cream was good for them than potato!). But make sure you eat potatoes with their skins on. Other excellent foods are peas (best source of manganese for vegetarians); bananas (high in potassium); mushrooms; spinach and other green leafy vegetables; nuts; lentils and beans. Foods such as these should make up at least half of your diet. Check out your diet using the following diet check.

DIET ANALYSIS

Many people would like to believe that as long as they take their vitamin supplements they can keep eating all the 'bad' foods that they love. But you can't rely on just diet, supplements or exercise alone to keep you healthy. All three are essential. Check out your diet check using the following Diet Check. Score one point for each question answered 'yes'. The maximum score is 20 and the minimum score is 0.

Diet check   Tick √ for YES

Do you add sugar to food or drink almost every day?   ____
Do you eat foods with added sugar almost every day?   ____
(read the labels carefully)
Do you add salt to your food?   ____
Do you drink more than one cup of coffee most days?   ____
Do you drink more than three cups of tea most days?   ____

Tick √ for YES

Do you smoke more than five cigarettes a week?	—
Do you drink more than 1oz (28g) of alcohol a day?	—
(one glass of wine, 1 pint or 600ml of beer, or one	—
measure of spirits)	
Do you take other non-medical drugs?	—
(e.g. cannabis etc.)	
Do you eat fried food (e.g. bacon and eggs, fish and	—
chips) more than twice a week?	
Do you eat processed 'fast food' more than twice	—
a week?	
Do you eat red meat more than twice a week?	—
Do you often eat foods containing additives and	—
preservatives?	
Do you eat chocolate or sweets more than	—
twice a week?	
Does less than a third of you diet consist of raw fruit	—
and vegetables?	
Do you drink less than 1/2 pint (300ml) of plain water	—
each day?	
Do you normally eat white rice, flour or bread rather	—
than wholegrain?	
Do you drink more than 3 pints (1.7 litres) of milk	—
a week?	
Do you eat more than three slices of bread a day,	—
on average?	
Are there some foods you feel 'addicted' to?	

Your Score

0 to 4 You're obviously a health-conscious individual and your minor indiscretions are unlikely to affect your health. Provided you supplement your diet with the right vitamins and minerals you can look forward to a long and healthy life.

5 to 9 You're on the right track, but must be stricter with yourself. Rather than 'giving up' your bad habits, set yourself easy experiments. For instance, for one month go without two of the foods or drinks you know are not good for you. Some you may then decide to have occasionally, while others you may find you go off. But be strict for one month - your cravings are only short-term 'withdrawal' symptoms. Aim to have your score below five within three months.

10 to 14 Your diet is not good and you will need to make some changes to be able to reach optimum health. But take it a step at a time. You should aim to have your score down to five within six months. Start by following the advice in this chapter. You will find that some of you bad dietary habits will change for the better as you find tasty alternatives. The 'bad habits' that remain should be dealt with one at a time. Remember that sugar, coffee and chocolate are all addictive. Your cravings will decrease after one month.

15 to 20 There is no way you can continue to eat like this and remain in good health. You are consuming far too much fat and refined foods. Follow the advice in this chapter very carefully and make gradual and permanent changes to your lifestyle. For instance, take two questions to which you answered 'yes' and make changes so that one month later you would answer 'no'. Keep doing this until your score is five or less. You may feel worse for the first two weeks, but within a month you'll feel the benefits.

Vitality Diet

One secret of a longer and healthier life is to eat foods high in vitamins and minerals. But this is not the only criterion for judging a food to be good. Good food should also be low in fat, salt and fast-releasing sugars, high in fibre, and high in alkaline-forming foods. Non-animal sources of protein are desirable. Such a diet will also be low in calories, but you won't have to count them, because your body will become increasingly efficient and will not crave extra food. Craving for food when you have eaten enough is often a craving for more nutrients, so foods providing 'empty' calories are out. The golden rules for a healthy diet are:

> Avoid sugar.
> Avoid refined carbohydrates, including white bread, biscuits, cakes and other refined food.
> Eat more beans, lentils and wholegrains.
> Eat more vegetables, raw or lightly cooked.
> Eat three pieces of fresh fruit a day.
> Avoid coffee, tea, cigarettes and limit alcohol.

The list below tells you which foods are good and bad from all these different points of view.

ALKALINE-FORMING FOODS all fresh fruit and vegetables; millet; almonds; brazil nuts; herb teas; yoghurt; bean sprouts.

ACID-FORMING FOODS beans; all meat and fish; grains; most nuts; seeds; milk produce; tea; coffee; chocolate; sugar; fats.

LOW FAT FOODS seafood; low fat yoghurt and cheese; skimmed milk; soya milk; tofu; beans; vegetables; fruit.

HIGH FAT FOODS meat; dairy produce, including butter, cheese and ice cream; margarine; vegetable oils.

NON-MEAT PROTEIN FOODS milk; cheese; yoghurt; eggs; beans; rice; lentils; nuts; seeds; tofu.

MEAT PROTEIN FOODS all meat, e.g. beef, pork, lamb; also chicken and fish.

SLOW-RELEASING SUGARS fresh fruit; unprocessed wholegrains, e.g. muesli; brown rice; lentils; beans.

FAST-RELEASING SUGARS white, brown and raw sugar; molasses; maple syrup; glucose, malt, honey and most syrups.

HIGH POTASSIUM FOODS fruit, including pineapples, grapes and bananas; vegetables; dandelion coffee; chicory coffee.

HIGH SODIUM FOODS salt, including sea salt; yeast extracts; all smoked fish; some cheeses; crisps; salted nuts; most canned foods; soya sauce.

UNREFINED FOODS nuts; seeds; wholegrains; wholemeal flour and bread; lentils; beans; brown rice.

REFINED FOODS white flour and bread; white, brown and raw sugar; white rice; processed and most packaged foods.

The following ideas and recipes will help you to change to a more healthy and enjoyable diet. As you become familiar with new foods (there are, for example, over twelve different kinds of beans), variety will never be a problem. Some suggestions are for 'instant' snacks when time is short; others are for proper meals. All are tried and tested and easy to make.

BREAKFASTS

Sugar Free Muesli
Choose 2oz dried fruit like prunes, figs and apricots, cover with water and simmer until soft. Add to a good quality sugar free muesli. Add a little soya milk to taste.

Fruit Breakfast
Have a large slice of melon, some grapes, some dried dates, figs or prunes. Adding a small handful of sesame and pumpkin seeds enriches this breakfast.

Breakfast Whizz
Liquidise a banana some strawberries and grapes together with a handful of nuts and seeds.

Fruit Milkshake
Liquidise peaches, strawberries or bananas (or any fruit you care to try) with ground almonds, dessicated coconut and some ice. Add milk and liquidise again.

Banana Yoghurt
Chop a banana into plain, unsweetened yoghurt. Mix in wheatgerm, sunflower seeds, coconut flakes or ground sesame seeds to taste.

Porridge
Place a small cup of porridge oats with 1.5 cups of water or milk into saucepan. Bring to boil and simmer for 5 minutes. Top with banana to sweeten or fruit of your choice.

Scrambled Eggs
Whisk 2 large eggs and a little parsley together. Gently melt .5 tsp of butter in small saucepan. Add eggs and cook gently, stirring with a fork until lightly set. Grill some wholemeal toast, top with scrambled egg and garnish with sliced grilled tomato.

QUICK LUNCHES

Jacket Potatoes with Chilli Bean Filling
Oven bake or microwave 1 large potato. Heat a small tin of kidney beans in chilli sauce and pile onto cooked potato. Serve with a generous helping of salad.

Jacket Potato, Crudites and Satay Sauce
Blend together 4tbsp peanut butter, 4tbsp tahini, 1tbsp lemon juice, 1 clove garlic and a little vegetable stock. Serve with a jacket potato and crudites - celery, carrot, cauliflower and peppers cut into sticks.

Three Bean Salad
8oz haricot beans tinned or dried. If dried soak overnight. Drain soak water. Cover with water and bring to boil. Continue boiling rapidly for 10 minutes. Simmer for 1 hour until soft. 8oz chick peas. (Follow same soak, boiling and cooking instructions as above.) 8oz green beans. While still warm add lemon and garlic dressing to cooked beans. Mix 1 tbsp of olive oil, rind of half a lemon, 2 tbsp of lemon juice and 1 crushed clove of garlic. Chill and serve.

Rainbow Root Salad
Grate carrots, parsnips and raw beetroot and mix with chopped parsley. Make an Island dressing by liquidising carrot, tomato, tofu, mayonnaise, ground almonds, Vecon, milk and grated nutmeg.

Garden Salad with Avocado Dressing
Mix lettuce, tomato, spring onion, brocolli, mangetout, courgette and herbs. For the dressing puree the avocado with a little lemon juice, a clove of garlic, and some vegetable stock.

Root Vegetable Salad with Tomato Juice Dressing
Shred carrot, beetroot, celeriac, parsnip or turnip and serve with sprouted alfalfa or mung seeds. For the dressing dissolve 1/2 teaspoon vegetable stock in a little water and stir in 1/2 teaspoon French mustard and add 1/4 pint tomato juice.

Chunky Vegetable Chowder
Chop some potato, onion, leek, carrot, celery and a clove of garlic. Simmer with some vegetable stock cube. Sprinkle with ground, toasted sesame and sunflower seeds.

Lentil Soup

Saute medium onion until soft, add 1tsp cumin and saute for half a minute, stirring all the time. Add a cup of split lentils with 2.5 pints of vegetable stock. Cook for 15-20 minutes, then blend, sieve if desired and serve the soup.

Open Sandwich

Top 2 slices of pumpernickel bread with 4oz. cottage cheese and alfalfa sprouts.

DINNERS

Marrow au Gratin

Heat 1 tbsp of olive oil and 2 tbsp of butter and melt. Saute a medium chopped onion and large garlic clove until transparent. Add four peeled and seeded tomatoes with 1 level tsp of tomato concentrate. Cook stirring constantly for a further 2 minutes. Add chopped; de-seeded, medium marrow, 2tbsp of finely chopped parsley and a generous pinch of oregano, with a little salt if desired then saute over a moderate heat until golden brown. Sprinkle with 2oz of grated cheese and 1oz of wholemeal bread crumbs and grill.

Winter Vegetable Casserole

Add 2 chopped onions, 1lb each of parsnips, carrot and potatoes and 1 red pepper to a pint of vegetable stock. Bring to boil and cook for 5 minutes. Add a tin of tomatoes and a tsp of parsley to stock. Mix 1 tbsp of potato flour in a little water and stir in carefully. Transfer to a baking dish and cook at 180$°$c for 50 minutes.

Chinese Vegetables

Saute 1 large onion with 1 tbsp of olive oil until soft. Add 1 tsp of ground ginger and stir for one minute. Add 2lb of frozen Chinese vegetables and cook until defrosted (or defrost in advance at room temperature or microwave). Add 4 tbsp of tamari soya sauce, 1lb of diced firm tofu and 1 tin of rinsed kidney beans. Bring to boil. then simmer for five minutes. Good served with brown rice or jacket potato.

Chick Pea Feast

Cook chick peas. Mix with chopped boiled eggs, flaked tuna fish and onion. Separately mix olive oil, vinegar, mustard, pepper, chopped parsley and chives and pour over chick peas. Serve hot.

Spicy Almond Couscous

Saute an onion. Add in sliced carrots, red pepper, courgettes and mushrooms. Add tomatoes, pepper or chilli sauce, almonds, raisins and water. Simmer for 20 minutes. Meanwhile pour boiling water over couscous and leave for 15 minutes.

Chestnut Hot Pot

Use fresh chestnuts, or soak dried chestnuts overnight. Add chestnuts, parsnips, swede, potato, turnip, bouillon powder and herbs to a pint of stock and simmer gently until chestnuts are cooked.

Fish Pie

Steam white fish, haddock and prawns. Combine with bechamel sauce made with wholemeal flour. Add in mushrooms, herbs and pepper. Top with mashed potatoes and bake for 30 minutes.

Spaghetti Napolitana

For sauce, saute an onion, garlic, carrots, green pepper and mushrooms. Add tomato puree, thyme and vegetable stock. Simmer and serve with wholemeal spaghetti.

Stuffed Peppers

Cook green peppers in boiling water for five minutes. Cut off top and scrape out seeds. Fry onion, garlic and tomatoes until softened. Add cooked rice, mushrooms, and stock. Simmer until cooked. Add egg, parsley and black pepper. Stuff peppers and bake in the oven.
* When sauteéing vegetables start with **very little** olive oil or butter, just to lightly cover the pan, then add 1-3 tbsps of water or vegetable stock to allow the ingredients to steam. This minimises the destruction of nutrients.

DESSERTS

Raspberry Surprise

Use 8oz of fresh, tinned or defrosted frozen raspberries, top with fromage frais, sweetened with a little honey, if desired.

Hunza Apricots with Cashew Cream

Soak 8oz of hunza apricots in boiling water until soft adding lemon verbena teabag to the soak water for extra flavour. Stone soaked apricots and replace with a hazelnut. To make cashew cream, simply grind 8oz of cashews in a blender until fine. Trickle in water until semi thick. Arrange apricots and cream in a sundae glass.

Dried Apricot Slice
Liquidise 6oz of dried apricots, 2oz of sultanas and 2oz of coconut and add to make a thick puree apple juice. Press firmly into a dish containing a layer of coconut, and sprinkle the top with more coconut. Chill and serve in wedges.

Baked Date and Apple
Core cooking apples and stuff with dates. Sprinkle with cinnamon and bake in an oven until soft.

Raspberry Sorbet
Freeze whole raspberries and bananas (this can be done with any fruit). Allow them to thaw for five minutes, then liquidise and serve immediately.

Apricot Whisk
Stew dried apricots until soft. Liquidise with vanilla essence, yoghurt and curd cheese. Whisk egg whites stiffly and fold into mixture.

DRINKS

Herb teas are both refreshing and relaxing. The number of different flavours available in convenient tea bags is so large that you could have a different drink every day for a month! I highly recommend that you experiment with the different varieties and find one that suits your taste. Some of the most delicious ones are mixtures with names such as Lemon Mist, Red Zinger, Emperor's Choice and Almond Sunset. Peppermint, rosehip, mixed fruit and lemon verbena come a close second, while Rooibosch ('red bush' - a common tea in Africa) is often a good starting point as it is most like Indian tea in flavour and can be taken with milk.

If you are a coffee drinker then some of the coffee substitutes may suit you better. Again the choice is large and you should not give up until you've tried them all! Dandelion coffee and chicory are both very high in potassium, chicory having the 'bitter' taste of coffee. Caro and Barleycup are both very popular and are good ones to try first. Decaffeinated coffee is one stage better than ordinary coffee, but no decaffeinated coffee has all the caffeine removed and it still contains two other stimulants present in coffee. Remember also that numerous chemicals are used in the decaffeinating process.

It is good to drink some pure water, or some diluted, unsweetened fruit juice every day. Remember - you are 65% water.

16
YOUR OPTIMUM SUPPLEMENT PROGRAMME

Your nutritional needs can be calculated by looking at your lifestyle, and the signs and symptoms associated with deficiency. In the sections that follow all you have to do is answer the questions as best as possible. You can then work out your 'score' out of 10 for each nutrient. If you score **5 or more** the chances are you are not optimally nourished for that nutrient, given your lifestyle. If you score **less than 5** the chances that you are deficient are small. Even if you have no associated symptoms of deficiency it is still wise to eat an optimal diet and take a high potency multivitamin and mineral supplement every day.

This system also takes your lifestyle into account. So, if you are very stressed or live in a polluted environment your optimal nutrient needs will be increased even if you are symtom free. In the second part of this chapter I will show you how to turn these scores into your optimum supplement programme.

If you are currently suffering from a diagnosed medical condition or are unsure about your needs it is best to see a nutrition consultant (see page 152).

SYMPTOM ANALYSIS

Underline each symptom that you often experience. Many symptoms occur more than once. This is because different nutrient deficiencies can cause them. Each symptom you <u>underline</u> scores 1 point. A **bold underlined** symptom scores 2 points. Notice that if you had all the symptoms, the maximum score for each nutrient is 10 points. Put your score for each nutrient in the box.

Vitamin Profile

<u>A</u>

Mouth ulcers
Poor night vision
Acne
Frequent colds or infections
Dry flaky skin
Dandruff
Thrush or cystitis
Diarrhoea

R · 0
Y · 0

Your score ▢

<u>C</u>

Frequent colds
Lack of energy
Frequent infections
Bleeding or tender gums
Easy bruising
Nose bleeds
Slow wound healing
Red pimples on skin

R · 0
Y · 2

Your score ▢

<u>D</u>

Rheumatism or arthritis *R*
Back ache *Y*
Tooth decay
Hair loss *Y*
Excessive sweating *Y*
Muscle cramps, or spasms
Joint pain or stiffness *Y* *2*
Lack of energy

R · 5
Y · 5

Your score ▢

<u>B1</u>

Tender muscles
Eye pains
Irritability *R*
Poor concentration *R*
'Prickly' legs *R*
Poor memory *R*
Stomach pains
Constipation
Tingling hands
Rapid heart beat

R · 4
Y · 4

Your score ▢

<u>E</u>

Lack of sex drive *R*
Exhaustion after light exercise *R*
Easy bruising
Slow wound healing
Varicose veins
Loss of muscle tone *R*
Infertility

R · 4
Y · 6

Your score ▢

<u>B2</u>

Burning or gritty eyes *Y*
Sensitivity to bright lights *R Y*
Sore tongue
Cataracts
Dull or oily hair
Eczema or dermatitis *Y R*
Split nails *Y*
Cracked lips

R – 5
Y – 6
1

Your score ▢

B3
Lack of energy
Diarrhoea
Insomnia R Y
Headaches or migraines
Poor memory R Y
Anxiety or tension R - S
Depression Y - S
Irritability
Bleeding or tender gums
Acne

Your score ☐

B12
Poor hair condition R
Eczema or dermatitis R Y
Mouth over sensitive to
hot or cold Y
Irritability R - 4
Anxiety or tension Y R Y - S
Lack of energy
Constipation Y
Tender or sore muscles
Pale skin

Your score ☐

B5
Muscle tremors or cramps R
Apathy R
Poor concentration R Y R - 6
Burning feet or tender heels Y - 3
Nausea or vomiting
Lack of energy
Exhaustion after light exercise R Y
Anxiety or tension R Y
Teeth grinding R

Your score ☐

Folic Acid
Eczema R Y
Cracked lips R
Prematurely greying hair R - S
Anxiety or tension R Y Y - 4
Poor memory R Y
Lack of energy
Depression R Y
Poor appetite
Stomach pains

Your score ☐

B6
Infrequent dream recall R Y
Water retention R R - 8
Tingling hands
Depression or nervousness R Y
Irritability R
Muscle tremors or cramps R
Lack of energy
Flaky skin

Your score ☐

Biotin
Dry skin
Poor hair condition R - S
Prematurely greying hair Y - 2
Tender or sore muscles
Poor appetite or nausea
Eczema or dermatitis R Y

Your score ☐

Essential Fatty Acid Profile

Linoleic & GLA
Dry, rough skin R
Dry eyes
Frequent infections
Poor memory R Y

Loss of hair or dandruff Y
Excessive thirst R R - 4
Poor wound healing Y - 3
PMS or breast pain Y
Infertility

Your score ☐

113

Mineral Profile

Calcium

R-6
4-2

Muscle cramps or tremors R
Insomnia or nervousness R
Joint pain or arthritis R
Tooth decay
High blood pressure

Your Score

Magnesium

R

R

Muscle tremors or spasms
Muscle weakness
Insomnia or nervousness 4
High blood pressure
Irregular heart beat 4
Constipation 4

R-5
4-5

Fits or convulsions
Hyperactivity 4
Depression 4

Your Score

Iron

Pale skin 4
Sore tongue
Fatigue or listlessness
Loss of appetite or nausea
Heavy periods or blood loss

R-0
4-2

Your Score

Zinc

Poor sense of taste or smell
**White marks on more than
two finger nails**
Frequent infections
Stretch marks R 4

R-2
4-3

Acne or greasy skin
Low fertility
Pale skin 4
Tendency to depression R 4
Poor appetite

Your Score

Manganese

Muscle twitches R 4
Childhood 'growing pains'

R-4
4-4

**Dizziness or poor sense of
balance** 4
Fits or convulsions
Sore knees

Your Score

Selenium

4 **Family history of cancer** R
Signs of premature aging
Cataracts
High blood pressure
Frequent infections

R-2
4-2

Your Score

Chromium

Excessive or cold sweats 4
Dizziness or irritability 4
after 6 hours without food
Need for frequent meals
Cold hands 4

R-2
4-6

Need for excessive sleep or
drowsiness during the day 4
Excessive thirst R
'Addicted' to sweet foods

Your Score

Now put all scores into the SYMPTOMS column of the chart
on page 118.

LIFESTYLE ANALYSIS

The following 'checks' allow you to adjust your nutrient needs according to aspects of your health and lifestyle. Again, answer the questions as best you can and work out your score. If your answer is 'sometimes' put YES. In most checks the maximum score is 10, scoring 1 point for each YES answer, unless otherwise specified. A score of 0-4 is a low score requiring no adjustment; a score of 5 or more is a high score requiring adjustment.

If you have a high score in any check, you will need to add the points shown in the chart on page 118 to your individual nutrient scores. The easiest way to do this is to highlight those columns that relate to you with a highlighter pen.

Some checks are either YES or NO. Again, if you answer YES adjust your individual nutrient score as shown in the chart on page 118.

Energy Check

Tick √ for YES

Do you need more than 8 hours sleep a night? ___

Are you rarely wide awake and rearing to go within 20 minutes of rising? ___

Do you need something to get you going in the morning, like a tea, coffee of cigarette? ___

Do you have tea, coffee, sugar containing foods or drinks, or cigarettes, at regular intervals during the day? ___

Do you often feel drowsy or sleepy during the day, or after meals? ___

Do you get dizzy or irritable if you haven't eaten for six hours? ___

Do you avoid exercise because you haven't got the energy? ___

Do you sweat a lot during the night or day or get excessively thirsty? ___

Do you sometimes lose concentration or does your mind go blank? ___

Is your energy less now than it used to be? ___

Your Score

Stress Check

Tick √ for YES   R

Is your energy less now than it used to be? —
Do you feel guilty when relaxing? —
Do you have a persistent need for recognition or achievement? —
Are you unclear about you goals in life? —
Are you especially competitive? —
Do you work harder than most? —
Do you easily become angry? —
Do you often do two or three tasks simultaneously? —
Do you become impatient if people or things hold you up? —
Do you have difficulty getting to sleep, sleep restlessly or wake up —
with your mind racing?

R - 7
Y - 5

Your Score

Exercise Check

R   Y

Do you take exercise that noticeably raises your heartbeat
for at least 20 minutes more than three times a week?

Does your job involve lots of walking, lifting or any
other vigorous activity?

Do you regularly play a sport? (football, squash, etc.)
Do you have any physically tiring hobbies?
(gardening, carpentry, etc.)
Do you consider yourself fit?

R - 0
Y - 0 .

Score 2 points for each YES answer.   Your Score

Immune Check

R

Do you get more than three colds a year? —
Do you find it hard to shift an infection (cold or otherwise)? —
Are you prone to thrush or cystitis? —
Do you generally take antibiotics twice or more each year? —
Is there a history of cancer in your family? —
Have you ever had any growths or lumps removed or biopsied? —
Do you have an inflammatory disease such as eczema, asthma or —
arthritis?
Do you suffer from hayfever? —
Do you suffer from allergy problems? —
Have you had a major personal loss in the last year? —

Your Score

Y - 4
R - 2

Pollution Check

Tick √ for YES

Do you live in a city or by a busy road? ___
Do you spend more than two hours a week in heavy traffic? ___
Do you exercise (job, cycle, play sports) by busy roads? ___
Do you smoke more than five cigarettes a day? ___
Do you live or work in a smoky atmosphere? ___
Do you buy foods exposed to exhaust fumes from busy roads? ___
Do you generally eat non-organic produce? ___
Do you drink more than 1 unit or oz of alcohol a day? ___
(one glass of wine, 1 pint of beer, or one measure of spirits) ___
Do you spend a considerable amount of time
in front of a TV or VDU screen? ___
Do you usually drink unfiltered tap water? ___

Your Score [ ]

Heart Check

Is your blood pressure above 140/90? ___
Is your pulse after 15 minutes' rest above 75? ___
Are you more than 14lb (7kg) over your ideal weight? ___
Do you smoke more than five cigarettes a day? ___
Do you do less than two hours of vigorous exercise (one hour if ___
you are over 50) a week?
Do you eat more than one tablespoonful of sugar each day? ___
Do you eat meat more than five times a week? ___
Do you usually add salt to your food? ___
Do you have more than two alcoholic drinks ___
(or units of alcohol) a day?
Is there a history of heart disease or diabetes in your family? ___

Your Score [ ]

Female Health Check

Are you trying to get pregnant, or are you pregnant, or are you breast-feeding? YES/NO

Do you regularly suffer from pre-menstrual syndrome, or have menopausal symptoms? YES/NO

Age Check

Are you under 14? (for YES, see page 121)
Are you 14 to 16? YES/NO
Are you over 60 (or post-menopausal)? YES/NO

117

NUTRIENT / SYMPTOMS	ENERGY	STRESS	EXERCISE	IMMUNE	POLLUTION	HEART	PREGNANT/ FEEDING	PMS/ MENOPAUSE	14-16	OVER 60
A (beta carotene)					2	1				1
D							1		1	1
E				1	1	1	1			
C	1	2	1	1	2	1				
B1	1	2	1							
B2	1	2	1							
B3	2	2	1				1			
B5	1	2	1							
B6	1	2	1	1			1	2	1	
B12							2			
Folic Acid							2			
Biotin							1		1	
GLA							2	2		1
Calcium		1		1	1	2		2		1
Magnesium	1	1	1	1				2		
Iron			1				1			
Zinc	1	1		2	2		2	2	1	
Manganese										
Selenium				1	1	1				
Chromium	2	1								

Figure 11a Calculating Your Nutrient Scores

YOUR TOTAL SCORE		UNITS	SCORE				YOUR IDEAL LEVEL
			0 - 4	5 - 6	7 - 8	9 or more	
=	A	iu	7,500	10,000	15,000	20,000	
=	D	iu	400	600	800	1,000	
=	E	iu	100	300	500	1,000	
=	C	mg	1,000	2,000	3,000	4,000	
=	B1	mg	25	50	75	100	
=	B2	mg	25	50	75	100	
=	B3	mg	50	75	100	150	
=	B5	mg	50	100	200	300	
=	B6	mg	50	100	200	250	
=	B12	mcg	5	10	50	100	
=	FA	mcg	50	100	200	400	
=	Biotin	mcg	50	100	150	200	
=	GLA	mg	-	150	225	300	
=	Cal	mg	150	300	450	600	
=	Mag	mg	75	150	225	300	
=	Iron	mg	10	15	20	25	
=	Zinc	mg	10	15	20	25	
=	Man	mg	2.5	5	10	15	
=	Sel	mcg	25	50	75	100	
=	Chro	mcg	20	50	100	200	

Figure 11b Converting Nutrient Scores into Supplement Levels

How to Work Out Your Optimum Nutrient Needs

From the Symptom Analysis you will have arrived at your basic score for each nutrient. These then need to be adjusted depending on the checks in the Lifestyle Analysis which add points to each nutrient. I recommend you highlight the columns that relate to you in the chart on page 118 and then add up the relevant scores in each row to arrive at your final score for each nutrient, which is the figure you put in the left hand column on page 119. The example below shows how to do this. The higher the score for any given nutrient the greater your need for that nutrient.

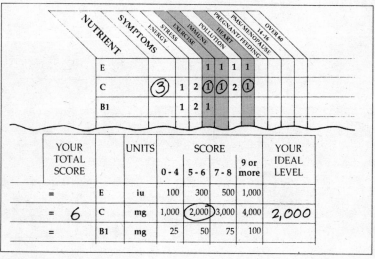

Figure 12 Example scoring

Turning Your Nutrient Scores Into Supplemental Levels

The score you've worked out still doesn't tell you how much you need to supplement. This is worked out using the adjacent chart on page 119. For example, if your vitamin C score was 6, your estimated ideal supplementary intake of vitamin C is 2,000mg per day. Now work out your supplemental levels for each nutrient.

Notice that if you score 0-4 on any nutrient I still recommend you to supplement a basic levels of these nutrients. These levels can easily be met by taking a good multivitamin and multimineral supplement every day. These levels are your supplementary needs, not your overall needs including diet. I have assumed that you will, improve your diet so that it provides a basic intake of these nutrients.

In other words these are you ideal needs in addition to a healthy diet. You will not get the same results from adding supplements to a poor diet.

Minerals other than those in the chart are generally sufficient in most people's diets and can be increased through dietary measures. Potassium, which balances sodium (salt), is best supplied through the diet by eating plenty of raw fruit and vegetables. Phosphorus deficiency is exceedingly rare and the mineral is contained in almost all supplements as calcium phosphate. Iodine deficiency is also extremely rare. Copper is frequently over-supplied in our diets and can be toxic. A wholefood diet is almost always sufficient in copper.

Scores for Children

There's a simple equation for working out approximate nutrient needs for children under 14. Take the weight of the child, in pounds, and divide by 100. (Alternatively, you can take the weight of the child in kilograms and divide by 50). Now multiply their supplemental levels by the division factor you've worked out to give their actual supplemental level.

So a child weighing 50lbs, divided by 100, gives 0.5. In our example, if the child scored 6 for vitamin C, this gives a supplemental level of 2,000mg. 2000mg multiplied by 0.5 gives 1,000mg. This is the child's approximate optimal intake of vitamin C.

How to Work Out Your Ideal Supplement Programme

In case you are wondering, you don't have to take 30 different supplements every day! Your needs can be compressed into four or five different supplements, each combining the nutrients above. The most common combinations are a multi-vitamin (containing vitamins A, B, C, D and E); and a multi-mineral for all the minerals. Vitamin C is usually taken separately since the basic optimum requirement of 1,000mg (1g) makes quite a large tablet without adding any more nutrients. Choosing the right formula is an art in itself. The next chapter will help you through the maze by showing you how to decipher the small print and read between the lines, so that you can devise a simple daily routine of vitamin supplements.

17

THE VALUE OF SAFE AND SENSIBLE SUPPLEMENTATION

Vitamin supplements can be very beneficial to our health in a stressful twentieth-century lifestyle. But not all supplements are the same. Analysis of a wide variety of multivitamin tablets to find out how much it would cost to get the basic optimum vitamin requirements produced a range between 20p and over £5 a day! And with so many supplements available, it's easy to become confused. For instance, if you're looking for a simple multivitamin preparation to meet the basic optimum requirements you have over 50 products to choose from.

So picking the right supplements is an art in itself. Unfortunately, not all supplements are true to their labels, so it is not always best to buy the cheapest. Reputable vitamin companies should give you a list of all the ingredients on the label.

Reading the label

Labelling laws vary from country to country, but many of the same principles stand. Depending on the ingredients, different laws apply and, since these change from time to time, many manufacturers are as confused as members of the public are! Figures 13a and 13b illustrate some of the problems you will confront when setting out to read a label. Figure 13a gives insufficient information, is misleading, shows dosages that are far too low and does not show any vitamins B6 or D, magnesium, chromium, manganese or selenium. The words used in the list of ingredients do not provide easy identification of the nutrients present and the fillers and binders - which make up more than 75 per cent of the tablets - are not described. The 'elemental' value of the minerals is not stated; nor is the amount of each nutrient per tablet. The form of vitamin E used is not stated: it could be mixed tocopherols, which are much less potent that d-alpha tocopherols. Ferrous fumarate can be a toxic form of iron. Finally, most people have too much copper already, so this should not be contained in a multivitamin unless there is ten times as much zinc, since copper is a zinc antagonist.

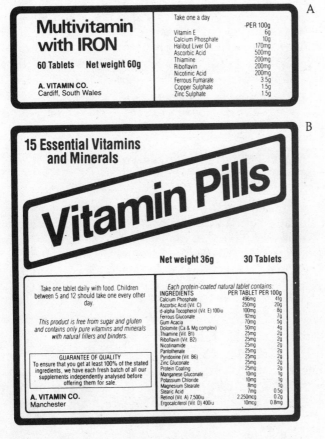

Figure 13 *What to Look For in a Supplement Label*

You ought not to find a multivitamin label as bad as this one! But it will give you some idea of what to look out for. Compare it with Figure 13b, where the dosages are correct, the chemical names for the different vitamins are given, and the filler (calcium phosphate) is listed. Directions for when and how to take the tablets are given, as well as extra information and a guarantee of quality. These are the things to go for when you are buying supplements: do not be misled by an attractive-looking label or a very cheap price, but do not pay too much either!

Active Ingredients

For all supplements the ingredients have to be listed in order of weight, starting with the ingredient present in the greatest quantity. This is often confusing since included in this list are the non-nutrient additives needed to make the tablet. For instance, in Figure 13b the first ingredient, calcium phosphate, is a 'filler'. In this case it does also provide nutritional benefit, so it is a good filler substance to use. Often the chemical name of the nutrient is used instead of the common vitamin code (for example, ergocalciferol for vitamin D).

The most confusing labels of all may give you only information like:

Cod Liver Oil tablets (750 capsules) Net Weight: 150g
Ingredients per 100g: Retinol 516mg

To find out how much vitamin A you would be getting you have to be a mathematician! If 750 capsules weigh 150g, 100g is equivalent to 500 capsules. Since 500 capsules therefore contain 516mg, each capsule contains 1.032mg or 1,032mcg of retinol (vitamin A). Converted to International Units (1iu = 0.34mcg) that's 3,000iu per capsule. Good vitamin companies keep you better informed than this.

Fillers and Binders

Tablets start off as powders. To get the bulk right 'fillers' are added. 'Binders' are added to give the mixture the right consistency and lubricants are also used. Only when this is done can the mixture be turned into small, uneven granules, which are then pressed into tablets under considerable force. Granulating allows the mixture to lock together, forming a solid mass. The tablet may then be coated with a 'protein coating' to protect it from deterioration and make it easier to swallow.

Unfortunately, many tablets also have colouring and flavouring added, as well as a sugar coating. For instance, many vitamin C tablets are made to look orange and taste sweet, since we associate vitamin C with oranges! Vitamin C is naturally almost white and certainly isn't sweet - and nor should your supplement be. The following fillers and binders are fine to use and some add extra nutritious properties to the tablet:

Dicalcium phosphate - a natural filler providing calcium and phosphate
Cellulose - a natural binder consisting of plant fibre
Alginic acid/sodium alginate - a natural binder from seaweed
Gum acacia/gum arabic - a natural vegetable gum
Calcium or magnesium stearate - a natural lubricant
Silica - a natural lubricant
Zein - a corn protein for coating the tablet
Brazil wax - a natural coating from palm trees

Many of the better tablets will also declare that the product is free from sugar and gluten. If you are allergic to milk or yeast do check that the tablets are also free from lactose (milk sugar) and yeast. Many B vitamins are derived from yeast, so you need to be careful. If in doubt, contact the company and ask for an 'independent assay' of the ingredients: good companies will supply this information. Sometimes glucose, fructose or dextrose is used to sweeten a tablet and yet the tablet still declares 'no sugar'. A small amount of fructose is the least evil if you're having difficulty enticing a child to take vitamins. Any other preservatives or flavouring agents should be avoided unless they are natural. For instance, pineapple essence is a natural additive.

If you are strictly vegan or vegetarian check the protein coating and the inclusion of stearates. These are often of animal origin, although they needn't be. Retinol (vitamin A) can either be synthesized or derived from animal source. Vitamin D can be synthesized, derived from sheep wool or from vegetable source. Companies do not have to state the source of the nutrients, just their chemical form.

Capsules Versus Tablets

Capsules are almost always made of gelatin, which is an animal product and therefore not suitable for vegetarians. Many capsules also contain a preservatives which stop the gelatin decaying or dissolving. I prefer not to take such preservatives and therefore avoid capsules unless I know their preservative free. Most vitamins can be provided as tablets. For instance, natural vitamin E comes in two forms: d-alpha tocopherol acetate (oil) or d-alpha tocopherol succinate (powder). Both are equally potent.

Natural Versus Synthetic

A great deal of nonsense has been said and written about the advantages of natural vitamins. First of all, many products claiming to be natural simply aren't. By law, a certain percentage of a product must be natural for the product to be declared 'natural'. The percentage varies from country to country. By careful wording some supplements sound natural but really aren't. For instance, 'vitamin C with rosehips' invariably means synthetic vitamin C with added rosehips, although it is often confused with vitamin C from rosehips. So which is better?

By definition, a synthetic vitamin must contain all the properties of the vitamin found in nature. If it doesn't then the chemists haven't done their job properly. This is the case with vitamin E. Natural d-alpha tocopherol succinate is 36 per cent more potent than the synthetic vitamin E called dl-alpha tocopherol (in this case the 'l' denotes the chemical difference). So natural vitamin E, usually derived from wheat germ or soya oil, is better.

However, synthetic vitamin C (ascorbic acid) has the same biological potency as the natural substance, according to Dr Linus Pauling, although chromatography and Kirlian photography have shown visible differences between the two. No one has yet shown that natural vitamin C is more potent or beneficial to take. Indeed, most vitamin C is synthesized by taking a 'natural' sugar, such as dextrose; a few chemical reactions later you have ascorbic acid. This is little different from the chemical reactions that take place in animals that convert sugar to vitamin C. Vitamin C derived from, say, acerola cherries - the most concentrated source - is also considerably bulkier and more expensive. Acerola is only 20 per cent vitamin C, so a 1,000mg tablet would be five times as large as a normal tablet and would cost you ten times as much!

It is true that vitamins derived from natural sources may contain an unknown element that increases their potency. Vitamin E, called d-alpha tocopherol, is found with other tocopherols, beta, gamma and delta tocopherol. So the inclusion of these with a measured amount of d-alpha tocopherol may be of benefit. Vitamin C is found in nature together with the bioflavanoids, active nutrients that appear to increase the potency of vitamin C, particularly in its capacity of strengthening the capillaries or tiny blood vessels. The best source of bioflavanoids is citrus fruit where it is found mainly in the pith, so the addition of citrus bioflavanoids to vitamin C tablets is one step closer to nature.

It is possible that yeast and rice bran, which are excellent sources of B vitamins, also contain unknown beneficial ingredients, so these vitamins are best supplied with yeast or rice bran. Brewer's yeast tablets or powder are far less efficient ways of taking B vitamins than B Complex vitamin supplements - one would have to eat pounds of yeast tablets to get optimum levels of B vitamins. However, watch out for yeast. Some people are allergic to it and if you react badly to any vitamin supplements it could be yeast causing the problem.

There are many other potentially helpful substances that may be provided with nutrients in a complex. Included here are co-enzymes that help to convert the nutrient into its active form. Vitamin B6 needs to be converted from pyridoxine to pyridoxal-5-phosphate before it becomes active in the body. The enzyme that does this is zinc dependent. For this reason a number of B6 supplements contain zinc. There are now supplements of pyridoxal-5-phosphate which should, theoretically, be more usable. Time will tell how much of an advantage these innovations will prove. But the key point is to make sure you get enough of each of the essential nutrients.

Elemental Minerals

Minerals in multivitamin and mineral tablets often omit the 'elemental' value of the compound, stating only the amount of the mineral compound. For instance, 100mg of zinc gluconate will provide only 10mg of zinc and 90mg of gluconate. Since it's the mineral you're after, check the figures carefully. If your supplement says 'zinc gluconate (providing 5mg zinc) 50mg' or 'zinc (as gluconate) 5mg' you're probably getting 5mg of zinc. Otherwise, you may have to contact the manufacturer for more detailed information. Most good companies declare this information either on the label or in literature that comes with the product.

When a mineral is attached to a compound such an an amino acid it is called 'chelated', from the Greek word for a claw. Chelated minerals are often absorbed much better and, in a sense, mimic what the body does normally. When we ingest a mineral it is normally

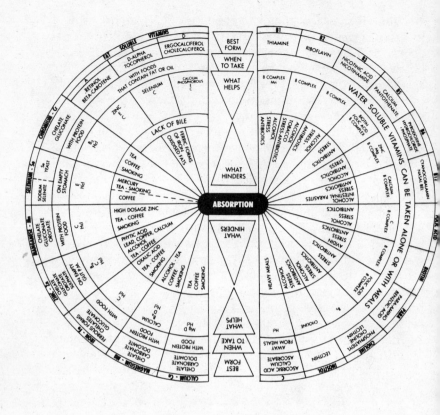

Figure 14 *Maximising Absorption of Vitamins and Minerals*

combined with an amino acid, a constituent of protein, to be absorbed. So minerals normally have to compete for amino acids - and not all of them win. By providing already chelated minerals absorption is far better.

Figure 14 shows you which forms of vitamins and minerals are best absorbed, and the factors that help, or hinder their absorption.

What is Sustained Release?

Some vitamins are called prolonged, sustained or time released, implying that the ingredients are not all made available for absorption in one go. This can be useful when taking large amounts of water-soluble vitamins such as B Complex or vitamin C. However, absorption depends also on the person and on the dosage. Some people are able to absorb and use 1,000mg of vitamin C taken in one dose; taking it in sustained release form would provide little benefit. However, if you take three 1,000mg tablets each day, sustained release would allow you to take them all in one go. Since sustained release vitamins are more expensive one has to weigh up the pros and cons. There is no point in having a sustained release fat-soluble vitamin, such a vitamins A, D or E, as these can be stored in the body.

Which Supplements Are Good Value?

For a supplement to be good value it must be well made, well formulated and well priced. The quality of manufacture is hard to assess unless you have an advanced chemistry laboratory in your back room! However, there are three simple tests you can do:

1 Are the stated number of tablets actually in the bottle? (We tested one company and found an average of 95 tablets instead of 100!)

2 Is the tablet coated all round and therefore easy to swallow? (Uncoated or badly coated tablets can break up or taste unpleasant.)

3 Does the label tell you everything you need to know? (The better the company the more information they will want to give you.)

Ideal Formulas

Every nutritionist has different ideas about the 'best' blend of vitamins and minerals in supplements, and this is reflected in the ever-growing range to choose from. The ideal formulation ultimately depends on your needs, but there are certain basic ones that act as building blocks for your Personal Health Programme. These are a multivitamin, a multimineral and a vitamin C tablet. These recommended formulas will cover the basic nutrient requirements for optimum health. Depending on your signs of deficiency you may also need to add extra B vitamins or individual minerals.

MULTIVITAMIN This should contain 7,500iu of A, 400iu of D, 100iu of E, 250mg of C and 50mg of B1, B2, B3, B5 and B6, 10mcg of B12, 50mcg of folic acid and biotin, plus PABA, choline and inositol.

MULTI-MINERAL This should provide 150mg of calcium, 75mg of magnesium, 10mg of iron, 10mg of zinc, 2.5mg of manganese, 20mcg of chromium and 25mcg of selenium.

VITAMIN C This should provide 1,000mg of vitamin C with at least 25mg of bioflavanoids.

How to Turn Your Nutrient Needs Into a Simple Supplement Programme

From your scores in the checks in Chapter 16, you will have worked out your optimum daily nutrient needs. If you scored less than five on each vitamin and mineral your needs are easily covered by this programme:

SUPPLEMENT	DAILY
Multivitamin	1
Multimineral	1
Vitamin C 1,000mg	1

If you scored five or more for vitamins A, D or E, you'll probably need to double the multivitamin. A score of seven or more on vitamin E will warrant a separate vitamin E supplement. If you scored seven or more on at least two B vitamins your best bet is to take one B Complex tablet per day. However, if you only scored high on B6, for example, adding a B6 supplement of the desired strength will be more practical. The same applies to vitamin C. If your optimum level is 2,000mg take two vitamin C tablets per day.

If you scored five or more for at least two minerals, you will probably meet your needs by doubling your multimineral intake. However, if only calcium and magnesium were deficient, these can be provided together in dolomite, a natural form of calcium and magnesium. If you are especially in need of chromium you may also require extra vitamin B3, so some manufacturers combine the two. The same is true for zinc and B6, so look out for these combined nutrients since they will save you money and decrease the number of tablets you take. If you have a weak immune system or a high pollution risk you may need more vitamin A, C, E, zinc and selenium. These are all anti-oxidant nutrients, immune and pollution protectors. Therefore they are often combined in supplements designed to meet these needs.

A Directory of Recommended Supplement Companies whose products meet these recommended levels of vitamin and mineral intake is given on page 153.

When Should You Take Vitamin Supplements?

Now that you've worked out what to take, you'll want to know when to take them. This depends not only on what is technically best, but also on your lifestyle. If taking supplements twice a day would mean that you'd forget the second lot, it is probably best for you to take them all at once! After all, nature supplies them all together, with a meal. Here are the 'ten commandments' of supplement taking:

1 Take vitamins and minerals 15 minutes before or after, or during a meal.

2 Take most of your supplements with your first meal of the day.

3 Don't take B vitamins late at night if you have difficulty sleeping.

4 Take multiminerals or dolomite tablets in the evening - these help you sleep.

5 If you're taking two or more B Complex or vitamin C tablets take one at each meal.

6 Don't take individual B vitamins unless you are also taking a general B Complex, perhaps in a multivitamin.

7 Don't take individual minerals unless you are also taking a general multimineral.

8 If you are anaemic (iron deficient) take extra iron with vitamin C. Avoid 'ferric' forms of iron.

9 If you know you are copper deficient take copper only with 10 times as much zinc, e.g. 0.5mg copper to 5mg zinc.

10 Always take your supplements every day. Irregular supplementation doesn't work.

Are There Any Side Effects?

The side effects of optimum nutrition are increased energy, mental alertness and a greater resistance to disease. In fact, a survey of supplement takers found that 79% noticed a definite improvement in energy, 66% felt more emotionally balanced, 60% had better memory and mental alertness, skin condition improved in 55% of people, and, overall, 61% had noticed a definite improvement in their well-being.[1] As long as you stick to the levels given in this book and don't take toxic levels, explained in Chapter 18, the only side effects are beneficial.

A very small number of people do, however, experience slight symptoms on starting a supplement programme. This may be because they take too many supplements with too little food, or perhaps because a supplement contains something that doesn't agree with them, for example, yeast. These problems are usually solved by stopping the supplements, then taking one only for four days, then adding another for the next four days and so on until all supplements are taken. This procedure will usually identify if there is a supplement that is causing a problem. More often than not the problem goes away.

Sometimes people feel worse before they feel better. Imagine if your body has been coping with the onslaught of pollution, poor diet, toxins and stimulants, and suddenly gets a wonderful diet and all the supplements it needs. This can lead to 'detoxification', the body cleansing itself. This is not a bad thing and usually subsides within a month. However, if you have inexplicable symptoms on starting a supplement programme or are suffering in any way see a nutrition consultant.

What Improvements in Health can I Expect?

Vitamins and minerals are not drugs, so you shouldn't expect an overnight improvement in your health. Most people experience definite improvement in health within three months. This is the shortest length of time that you should experiment with a supplement programme. The earliest noticeable health changes are increased energy, mental alertness and emotional stability and improvements in the condition of the skin. Your health will continue to improve as long as you are following the right programme. If you do not experience any noticeable improvement in three months, it is best to see a nutrition consultant.

How Often Should I Reassess My Needs?

Certainly at the beginning your needs will change and a reassessment every three months is sensible. Your nutrient needs should decrease as you get healthier. Remember, you need optimum nutrition most when you are stressed. So when the emergencies occur, or you're working especially hard, make doubly sure that you eat well and take your supplements every day.

18

THE MYTH OF
TOXICITY

Recently there has been a proliferation of reports in the popular press that vitamins, at least in the levels found in some supplements, might be doing you harm rather than good. Particularly under the spotlight are vitamin A, claimed to be toxic and potentially harmful during pregnancy, B6 claimed to damage the nervous system, and vitamin C claimed, in large doses, to contribute to the formation of kidney stones. Can these claims be substantiated and if so, how much is too much?

Your ideal intake of vitamins depends upon your viewpoint and your condition. Some people believe that the 'ideal' intake is the level that prevents obvious deficiency signs. The RDA's are considered, on the whole, to cover these needs. Other people, including myself, believe that the ideal intake of a vitamin is the level that promotes the best possible health, complete absence of any early warning signs of deficiency, and helps enzymes dependent on vitamins, function at their peak, as determined by biochemical tests. These 'optimum' levels are often 50 to 100 times greater than RDA levels. But even these levels often fall below the level shown to have a therapeutic effect on specific conditions. For example, the US RDA for vitamin C is 60mg, the optimum level is around 1,000mg, and the level shown to have therapeutic effect in the treatment of cancer is in the region of 10,000mg.

The basic, ideal and therapeutic levels vary considerably for each individual depending on their age, sex, health and numerous other factors. Therefore it is to be expected that the level of a vitamin that would induce signs of toxicity also vary considerably. In this chapter I have erred on the side of caution by listing the levels that may induce toxicity in a small percentage of people, both if taken over a short period of time (up to one month), and over a long period of time (three months to three years), and indicated if the symptoms persist or go away once the high level is reduced.

The general conclusion from a survey of the results of over one hundred research papers in major scientific journals is that for the majority of vitamins, with the exception of vitamin A and D, levels 100 times greater than the RDA are likely to be safe for long-term ingestion. **In practical terms, this means that the chances of having a toxic reaction to even the higher dose supplements available in health food shops, is extremely unlikely unless you take a considerably greater number of tablets than recommended.** This is broadly consistent with the absence of public health record of deaths attributed to nutritional supplements. For example, a survey of Local Poison Control Centers in the US between the years 1983 and 1987 listed 1,182 fatalities results from pharmaceutical drugs, and not one fatality resulting from a vitamin supplement. In Britain, I have been unable to find any death attributable to vitamin supplemention in the last decade as compared to thousands of deaths per year attributable to pharmaceutical drugs.

Vitamin A
Vitamin A comes in two forms: the animal form, retinol, which stores in the body; and the vegetable form, beta-carotene, which is converted into retinol, unless body levels are already high. Beta-carotene is therefore not considered toxic, with the exception that excessive intake can cause a reversible yellowing of the skin.

There are a number of incidences of adverse reactions to retinol, usually from intakes of 500,000ius or more over a considerable length of time. The symptoms include peeling and redness of the skin, disturbed hair growth, lack of appetite and vomiting. According to Dr John Marks, medical director at Girton College, University of Cambridge, "toxic reactions have been extremely rare below 30,000ius...daily administration in adults up to about 50,000ius would appear to be safe." This is consistent with estimates of the intake of 40,000ius of vitamin A that our ancestors would have eaten in a more tropical environment, although a large part of this would have come from beta-carotene.

A number of cases of toxicity and possibly associated birth defects have been reported for a synthetic relative of vitamin A, isotretinoin, sold as the drug Roaccutane. These reports of birth defects have been wrongly extended to natural vitamin A. Five cases of birth defects have been reported in women taking large amounts of retinol (25,000 to 500,000ius per day) however no clear cause and effect relationship has ever been established in any of these cases. Other studies have shown that women who supplement their diet with multivitamins including vitamin A usually at a level of 7,500 to 25,000iu have a lower incidence of birth defects. In view of the unlikely possibility that retinol, in large amounts, could induce birth defects, it may be wise for women of a child bearing age to supplement no more than 10,000ius of retinol. The same caution does not apply to beta-carotene.[1-19]

Vitamin D

Of all the vitamins vitamin D is the most likely to cause toxic reactions. Vitamin D encourages calcium absorption and excessive intake can lead to calcification of soft tissue. However the levels that create this effect are certainly in excess of 10,000ius and probably more like 50,000ius. A daily intake not exceeding 2,000ius for adults and 1,000ius for children is generally considered to be safe.[20-38]

Vitamin E

Vitamin E has been well researched for toxicity. A review of 216 trials of high dose vitamin E in 10,000 patients showed that daily doses of 3,000ius for up to eleven years and 55,000ius for a few months had no detrimental effect. However, adverse reactions have occasionally been reported at lower levels of 2,000ius, especially in children. Vitamin E appears to potentiate the anti-clotting effects of the drug Warfarin, and therefore high levels are not recommended for those on this drug. High levels are also best avoided by those suffering from rheumatic fever. People with high blood pressure are also encouraged to start at a low level of supplementation, say 100iu per day, adding 100iu per month until they reach their desired intake. A daily intake of up to 1,500iu is considered safe.

Vitamin C

Vitamin C is water soluble and therefore excess is readily excreted from the body. RDA's vary considerably from country to country. A general consensus, based on up to date research, is that 1000mg a day represents a good basic intake. The optimal intake is probably between 1,000 and 3,000mg a day. A number of studies have investigated the effects of vitamin C on specific diseases using over 10,000mg a day. The recommendation of these high levels have attracted controversy and allegations that vitamin C can cause kidney stone formation, interferes with B12 absorption, and causes a 'rebound scurvy' when supplementation is stopped. All of these allegations have been shown to be without substance. The only adverse effect of taking large amounts of vitamin C is that it can have a laxative effect. There is some tentative evidence that vitamin C might increase the potency of the contraceptive pill. This has yet to be substantiated and anyway is not a toxic effect of vitamin C, but a point of caution for those taking oral contraception. Generally, supplementing up to 5,000mg of vitamin C can be considered safe.[39-54]

B Vitamins

B vitamins are water soluble and excess is readily excreted from the body via the urine. Hence they are generally of very low toxicity. Thiamin (B1), riboflavin (B2), pantothenic acid (B5), B12 and biotin show no sign of toxicity at levels of at least 100 times the US RDA. Vitamin B3, in the form of niacin, causes a blushing sensation at levels of 75mg or more. This is part of its natural action and therefore is not a toxic effect. According to Dr John Marks, director of medical studies at Girton College, Cambridge, "doses of 200mg to 10g daily have been used therapeutically to lower blood cholesterol levels under medical control for periods of up to ten years or more, and though some reactions have occurred at these very high dosages, they have rapidly responded to cessation of therapy, and have often cleared even when therapy has been continued." Levels of up to 2,000mg per day on a continuous-basis are considered safe, although they will induce blushing (vasodilation). Sustained release niacin, however, may have potential toxicity at lower doses and is best avoided. [55-64]

Vitamin B6 has been extensively tested for toxicity by a number of research groups including the US government Food and Drug Administration who concluded "in man, side effects were not encountered with daily administration of 50-200mg over periods of months". Most of the reports of low dose B6 causing nerve damage appear to be based on one well documented case of a woman who increased her B6 intake from supplements from 500mg to 5,000mg over a period of two years, and developed muscle weakness and pain, attributed to nerve damage. One researcher, investigating seven cases of people taking 2,000 to 5,000mg a day of B6 for considerable lengths of time said that "substantial improvement occurred in all cases in the months after withdrawal of pyridoxine, usually with improvement in gait and less discomfort in the extremities, but in some patients, residual neurological discomfort remained." In rats, daily doses of 600mg/kg, equivalent to 38,000mg a day in a ten stone person, by injection, caused nerve damage. Deficiency of vitamin B6 induces the same symptoms. The likely explanation for this is that pyridoxine, in order to become active in the body where it helps enzymes to work, must be converted to pyridoxal phosphate. By saturating the body with excessive amounts of pyridoxine, this conversion doesn't take place and enzymes become saturated with simple pyridoxine and hence don't work properly. The excess of B6 may, in fact, induce effectively B6 deficiency symptoms. Since zinc is required for the conversion of pyridoxine to pyridoxal phosphate, taking B6 with zinc is likely to reduce its toxicity. In any event a daily intake of up to 200mg on a continuous basis is generally considered safe.55-78

Minerals

As with vitamins, myths abound concerning the danger of minerals, their essentiality and the need for supplements. Selenium, chromium and germanium have all been described in newspapers as 'poisons'. Zinc supplementation gets its fair share of criticism while others consider we could all do with a little extra. Likewise, calcium supplementation has been frowned upon as a potential cause of kidney stones, gall stones and calcium deposits in joints. Fact or fiction?

Minerals tend to be divided into two families. The 'macro' minerals calcium, magnesium, phosphorus, potassium and sodium, of which we need a relatively large amount each day to stay healthy - and the 'micro' or trace minerals, iron, zinc, copper, chromium, manganese and selenium. All these minerals are known to be essential for health. Other trace minerals such as molybdenum, boron, vanadium and germanium have some of the properties required for essentiality but have yet to be conclusively proven to be essential.

Some minerals are used for 'building material', for example calcium, others are used for their electrolyte properties in nerve and muscle function, such as sodium and potassium. But the main role of minerals is, like many vitamins, as co-factors for enzymes. Enzymes are the keys of life because they turn one substance into another. For example, they break down protein into amino acids ready for absorption and then rebuild protein to make body cells. The mineral co-factor is like the missing cog in the machine. No co-factor - no enzyme function. It's as simple as that.

The safety of minerals depends on three factors. Firstly, the amount. All minerals show toxicity at exceedingly high doses. Secondly, the form. Trivalent chromium, for example, is essential, while hexavalent chromium (found in neither foods nor supplements) is very toxic. Thirdly, the balance with other minerals in the diet. Iron supplementation can induce zinc deficiency since it is a zinc antagonist. The reason for this antagonism is that many minerals are atomically very similar to each other. They're just different sizes of cogs. So if you lack one mineral but take in an excess of another similar mineral it can interfere with enzyme function, speeding up or slowing down or simply blocking an enzyme from working.

In view of these factors the levels I have given as safe for long term ingestion presuppose that other essential minerals are also adequately supplied. Larger amounts than those stated may also be safe for short term ingestion, particularly for people with certain illnesses which result in an extra requirement for a mineral. Selenium requirement, for example, is thought to increase in certain types of cancer.

Calcium
Calcium comes in many forms, the best absorbed of which include calcium ascorbate, amino acid chelate, gluconate, orotate and carbonate. In normal, healthy people there is little danger of toxicity since the body excretes excessive amounts. Some cultures consume in excess of 2g a day from diet alone, so this amount is certainly considered safe. 3.6g per day is used to treat calcium deficiency disorders. Problems of excessive calcium arise from other factors such as excessive vitamin D intake (above 25,000ius per day), parathyroid or kidney disorders. Calcium interacts with magnesium and phosphorus, therefore calcium supplementation should only be given to those with an adequate magnesium and phosphorus intake, or also supplementing these elements. Phosphorus is rarely deficient while magnesium deficiency is quite common. The ideal calcium/phosphorus ratio is probably 2:1. Less than 1:2 is not desirable. The ideal calcium/magnesium ratio is probably 3:2.

Magnesium

Magnesium comes in many forms, the best absorbed of which include magnesium aspartate, amino acid chelate, gluconate, orotate and carbonate. Toxic effects of magnesium include flushing of the skin, thirst, low blood pressure, loss of reflexes and respiratory depression. Toxicity is only likely to occur in those with kidney disease taking magnesium supplements. For normal, healthy adults a daily intake of up to 1,000 mg is considered safe. Magnesium interacts with calcium, therefore magnesium supplements should only be given to those with adequate calcium intake, or supplementing calcium. The ideal magnesium/calcium ratio is probably 2:3 and, in cases of magnesium deficiency 1:1.

Iron

Iron is one of the most frequently deficient minerals. At least 6 per cent of women in the UK get below the RDA from their diets. Iron comes in many different forms, the best absorbed of which include ferrous aspartate, amino acid chelate, succinate, lactate and gluconate. (Ferric forms of iron are not required.) Ferrous sulphate induces symptoms of toxicity in animals at lower levels than these forms. As little as 3g of ferrous sulphate can cause death in an infant, compared to 12g for an adult. Therefore supplements containing a significant amount of iron should be kept in a child proof container away from children. Iron is stored in the body and therefore toxicity can result from long-term excess intake, producing haemosiderosis, a generalised deposition of iron within body tissue, or haemochromatosis, normally a hereditary condition resulting in cirrhosis of the liver, bronze pigmentation of the skin, diabetes, arthritis and heart abnormalities. Both conditions are extremely rare as a result of dietary intake. 50mg a day is generally considered safe.

Iron is antagonistic to many other trace minerals including zinc which is commonly deficient, especially among pregnant and lactating women. Therefore extra iron should not be supplemented without ensuring adequate zinc status or supplementing zinc. The normal requirement for zinc and iron is approximately equal.[79-88]

Zinc

Zinc is one of the most thoroughly researched and commonly deficient minerals. About a thousand papers are published each year indicating its value for a variety of conditions. The best absorbed forms of zinc include zinc picolinate, amino acid chelate, citrate and gluconate. Zinc supplementation is relatively non-toxic. In doses of 2,000mg symptoms of nausea, vomiting, fever and severe anaemia have been reported. Small amounts of zinc, particularly in the form of zinc sulphate, can act as an irritant in the digestive tract when taken on an empty stomach. There is also some evidence that zinc, at levels of 300mg per day, may impair rather than improve immune function. It is generally considered safe to supplement up to 50mg per day.

Zinc is an iron, manganese and copper antagonist, therefore an adequate intake of these minerals is advisable if large amounts of zinc are taken over a long period of time. Manganese is very poorly absorbed and therefore it is generally advisable to supplement half as much manganese as zinc if more than 20mg of zinc is supplemented per day. The normal requirement for zinc is about ten times that of copper. Since the average intake of copper for those on a healthy diet is in the order of 2mg, those supplementing more than 20mg of zinc may be advised to add 1mg of copper for each additional 10mg of zinc. It is also best to ensure that at least 12mg of iron is supplemented when taking more than 20mg of zinc.[89-101]

Copper
Copper deficiency is quite rare, probably because we receive it from drinking water as well as from unrefined foods. The best absorbed forms of copper include copper amino acid chelate and gluconate. Requirements are low (2mg per day) and only 5mg a day are required to correct deficiency. Copper toxicity does occur, mainly due to excessive intake as a result of copper plumbing. Copper is also a strong antagonist of zinc and for this reason it is advisable not to supplement more than 2mg or a tenth of one's intake of zinc. Copper also depletes manganese.

Manganese
Only 2 to 5 per cent of dietary manganese is absorbed and therefore larger intakes have a small effect on overall body levels. The better forms for absorption include amino acid chelate and gluconate There is some evidence that vitamin C may help the absorption of manganese. In animals it is one of the least toxic of all trace elements. Toxicity has never been reported in man. A daily intake of up to 50mg is considered safe. Excessive zinc or copper intake interferes with manganese uptake.

VITAMINS	OPTIMUM RANGE	MAXIMUM SAFETY LEVEL
A	7,500 - 20,000 iu	33,333 iu*
D	400 - 1,000 iu	2,000 iu
E	100 - 1,000 iu	1500 iu
C	1,000 - 4,000 mg	6,000 mg
B1	25 -100 mg	140 mg
B2	25 - 100 mg	160 mg
B3	50 - 150 mg	180 mg
B5	50 - 300 mg	400 mg
B6	50 - 250 mg	300 mg
B12	5 - 100 mcg	300 mcg
Folic Acid	50 - 400 mcg	2,000 mcg
Biotin	50 - 200 mcg	10,000 mcg

* For women of child-bearing age the maximum safety level for long term use is 10,000 iu

MINERALS		
Calcium	400 - 800 mg	3,000 mg
Magnesium	300 - 500 mg	1,000 mg
Iron	10 - 25 mg	50 mg
Zinc	15 - 30 mg	50 mg
Copper	1 - 3 mg	5 mg
Manganese	5 - 25 mg	100 mg
Selenium	50 - 250 mcg	500 mcg
Chromium	50 - 250 mcg	500 mcg

Figure 15 *Vitamins and Minerals - How Much Is Safe?*

Selenium

Selenium is required in very small amounts of 25 to 200mcg per day. It comes in two forms: organic such as selenomethionine or selenocystine, sometimes in the form of selenium yeast; and inorganic sodium selenite. The inorganic form is more toxic, with toxicity occurring at levels of 1,000mcg or more. The organic forms show toxicity above 2,000mcg. No toxicity has been reported with either form at intakes of 750mcg. An intake of up to 500mcg for an adult is generally considered safe. In view of the relatively small difference between a beneficial and a detrimental intake, selenium should also be kept out of reach of children.

Chromium

Chromium is found in two forms in nature-hexavalent and trivalent. Hexavalent chromium is much more toxic, however it is neither found in food nor supplements so contamination can only occur from occupational exposure. The better absorbed forms of chromium are picolinate and amino acid chelate. Trivalent chromium has a very low toxicity partly because so little is absorbed. Cats show signs of toxicity at 1,000mg per day. An intake of up to 500mcg is certainly considered safe.

Even the highest levels I have recommended in this book are well within maximum safety levels.

19
A - Z OF OPTIMUM NUTRITION FOR COMMON AILMENTS

While there is no substitute for individual assessment of nutrient needs, the following advice may be helpful. Many of the conditions are quite serious and you would be wise to follow these programmes under the supervision of your doctor or nutrition consultant. The supplements recommended are for adults, based on the formulas given in Chapter 17. Since dosage is crucial it is best to get supplements close to these formulas.

Acne
Acne is most prevalent among teenage boys and girls and the hormonal changes that take place at this age are certainly at the root of many skin problems. These changes cause the sebaceous glands to produce too much sebum, which blocks up the skin pores and makes them more likely to get infected. Optimum nutrition helps by balancing hormones as well as reducing the risk of infection. The most important nutrients are vitamins A, B Complex (especially B6), C and E and zinc. Good diet and cleanliness are essential.
DIET ADVICE Follow an optimum diet and drink plenty of water. Sulphur-rich foods such as eggs, onions and garlic are also helpful. Avoid sugar, cigarettes, frying and high fat foods.

SUPPLEMENTS 1 X Multi-vitamin; 1 x B Complex;
2 x Vitamin C 1,000mg; 1 x Vitamin B6 100mg
Zinc 10mg; 1 x Vitamin E 500iu

Alcohol Dependence

Alcohol dependence is particularly high among high histamine people, and may in part be a way of coping with the excess energy the high histamine person produces. B vitamins, especially B1, B2, B3 and B6, are destroyed by alcohol, which primarily affects the liver and nervous system. Vitamins A and C help protect the liver. A very alkaline diet reduces craving for alcohol. Emotional problems almost always underlie drinking problems.

DIET ADVICE Follow the vitality diet and eat plenty of wholegrains, beans and lentils. Drink plenty of water. Often, sugar addiction is substituted for alcohol, which is a different form of sugar, so sugar is also best avoided. Eat frequent meals containing some protein foods such as nuts, seeds, fish, chicken, eggs or milk produce.

SUPPLEMENTS 2 X Multi-vitamin; 1 x Multi-mineral
3 x Vitamin C 1,000mg; 1 x Vitamin B6 100mg; Zinc 10mg
3 x Dolomite

Allergies

Allergy is a word that often invokes connotations beyond its original meaning. An allergy is an intolerance to a particular substance. We have an intolerance to coffee, for example, in that large amounts produce symptoms. Some people have more pronounced symptoms even to simple foods like wheat or milk. Since an allergy is like an addiction, it is often the foods one is most 'addicted' to that are suspect. If you suspect that you might have allergies but do not know what they are, it is best to see a nutrition consultant or an allergy specialist.

DIET ADVICE Follow the vitality diet, being careful to avoid the substances to which you react. After two months you my be able to reintroduce these every fourth day without having a reaction. Eventually you may be able to tolerate your allergens in small amounts on a daily basis.

SUPPLEMENTS 2 x Multi-vitamin; 3 x Vitamin C 1,000mg
3 x Vitamin B6 100mg; 1 x zinc 10mg; 3 x Dolomite
2 x Manganese 10mg

Arthritis

There are two major forms of arthritis and many different causes for both. Osteoarthritis, more common in the elderly, describes a condition in which the cartilage in the joints wears away, inducing pain and stiffness mainly in weight-bearing joints. Rheumatoid arthritis affects the whole body, not just certain joints. Once more the cartilage is destroyed and replaced with scar tissue, which can eventually cause the joints to fuse together. Nutritionally speaking, the primary means to avoid these conditions is to provide support for the endocrine glands that are involved in proper utilisation of calcium, and the immune system in the case of arthritis. Vitamins C, B3, B5, B6 and D, calcium and magnesium are particularly important. Also associated with arthritic conditions are excesses or deficiencies of iron and copper and possibly manganese, all of which are involved in cartilage formation.

DIET ADVICE Follow the vitality diet and be sure to avoid adrenal stimulants such as tea, coffee, sugar, refined carbohydrates such as biscuits and cakes, salt, cigarettes and alcohol - many arthritic sufferers have eaten excesses of these in the past. Over-stressed people are also more likely to get rheumatoid arthritis. Drink plenty of water and herb teas.

SUPPLEMENTS 1 x Multi-vitamin; 1 x B Complex;
1 x Vitamin C 1,000mg; 2 x Multi-mineral;
2 x Vitamin B5 (Pantothenic acid) 250mg

Asthma

Asthma affects the lungs and respiration and is characterised by difficulty in breathing and frequent coughing. Often asthma attacks are brought on by an allergic reaction, stressful event or changes in environmental conditions like the weather or a smoky atmosphere. Vitamin A helps protect the lining of the lungs, while vitamin C helps to detoxify environmental toxins. However, for some people the cause of this condition may lie in hormonal imbalances.

DIET ADVICE Follow the vitality diet and see a nutrition consultant if you suspect that you may have some allergies.

SUPPLEMENTS
2 x Multivitamin; 2 x Vitamin C 1,000mg
1 x B Complex; 1 x Multimineral

Constipation

Contrary to popular belief one should empty one's bowels not once but twice a day. A healthy stool should break up easily and be no strain to pass. By these criteria a large majority of people suffer from constipation. A high fibre diet will help, as will a reduction in meat and milk produce. Exercise is also crucial as it strengthens the abdominal muscles. Vitamins B1 and E help to strengthen these muscles, and vitamin C may also loosen the bowels.

DIET ADVICE Follow the vitality diet with particular reference to eating high fibre foods. Drink at least one pint (600ml) of water a day, preferably between meals. Reduce your consumption of meat and milk produce.

SUPPLEMENTS

1 x Multivitamin; 1 x Multimineral; 2 x Vitamin C 1,000mg
1 x B Complex; 1 x Vitamin E 500iu

Diabetes and Hypoglycaemia

Diabetes is sub-divided into child-onset diabetes and adult-onset diabetes, both being conditions of high blood sugar. Hypoglycaemia, or low blood sugar, often precedes adult-onset diabetes. Child-onset diabetes is a total failure to make insulin. Together, the two conditions are disease of glucose intolerance. Ensuring the proper production of adrenal hormones, insulin and 'glucose tolerance factor' from the liver is fundamental for all forms of glucose intolerance. Particularly important therefore are vitamins C, B3, B5 and B6, zinc and chromium. People with diabetes must always seek medical advice, and discuss any proposed changes in their diet with a doctor.

DIET ADVICE Follow the vitality diet with the following modifications: eat small, frequent meals containing protein or complex carbohydrates (nuts, seeds, wholegrains, fish, chicken, eggs, cheese, beans, lentils); avoid all sugar and forms of concentrated sweetness, such as concentrated fruit juice, and even excesses of fruit or dried fruit. Also avoid excessive tea, coffee, alcohol and cigarettes.

SUPPLEMENTS 1 x Multivitamin; 2 x Vitamin C 1,000mg;
2 x Multimineral; 1 Vitamin B3 100mg; 1 x chromium 100mcg;
1 x B Complex

Eczema

Eczema is a skin condition in which the skin becomes scaly and itchy; it can crack and be very sore. Although the mechanism is unknown, optimum nutrition does usually help this condition. Vitamins A and C strengthen the skin, while vitamin E and zinc improve healing. When there is no open wound, vitamin E oil can help to heal the skin.

DIET ADVICE Follow the vitality diet. Test for likely allergies, including the effects of metals from watches and jewellry.

SUPPLEMENTS 1 x Multivitamin; 1 x Vitamin A 7,500iu
1 x B Complex; 1 x Vitamin E 500iu; 1 x Vitamin B6 100mg
1 x Zinc 10mg; 2 x Vitamin C 1,000mg; 1 x GLA
(gamma linolenic acid) 150mg

Hypertension (High Blood Pressure)

Hypertension (high blood pressure) atherosclerosis and arteriosclerosis usually go together. Arteriosclerosis means hardening of the arteries; atherosclerosis means narrowing of the arteries due to fatty deposits. Most of us have some degree of both. When the condition becomes more pronounced, blood pressure begins to increase. Vitamins A, C and E and selenium help prevent the cellular damage that may underlie these problems.

DIET ADVICE Follow the vitality diet strictly. Avoid sugar, salt, high fat foods, coffee and excess alcohol. Take plenty of exercise within your capacity and do not smoke.

SUPPLEMENTS 1 x Multivitamin; 1 x B Complex
3 x Vitamin C 1,000mg; 1 x Vitamin E 500iu
1 x Multimineral; 1 x Selenium 100mcg
1 x Vitamin B6 100mg; 1 x Zinc 10mg; I x EPA 360mg

Indigestion

Indigestion can be caused by many different factors including too little hydrochloric acid production in the stomach. In most cases, the symptoms of indigestion can be helped by following the principles of optimum nutrition; in some cases, additional enzymes are needed.

DIET ADVICE Follow an optimum diet, having as much alkaline forming foods as possible.

SUPPLEMENTS 1 x Multivitamin; 1 x Vitamin C 1,000mg
1 x B Complex; 1 x Multimineral; 3 x Dolomite
1 x Digestive enzymes with each meal.

Infertility

Infertility is more common in women than men, although in 30 per cent of couples who have difficulty conceiving, it is due to the man. Vitamins E and B6, and zinc are important for both sexes, and C is important for men. Also important are essential fatty acids.

DIET ADVICE Follow an optimum diet. Essential fatty acids are found in cold-pressed oils.

SUPPLEMENTS 1 x Multivitamin; 1 x Vitamin E 500iu 1 x B Complex; 2 x Vitamin C 1,000mg; 1 x Vitamin B6 100 mg; 1 x Zinc 20mg

Insomnia

For some sufferers the major problem of insomnia is waking up in the middle of the night, for others it's not getting to sleep in the first place. Both can be the result on the nervous system of poor nutrition or too much stress and anxiety. Calcium and magnesium have a tranquillising effect as does vitamin B6. Tryptophan, a constituent of protein, has the strongest tranquillising effect and if taken in doses of 1,000mg to 3,000mg, it is highly effective for insomnia. It takes about an hour to work and remains effective for up to four hours. While tryptophan is non-addictive and has no known side-effects, its regular use is not recommended - it is better to adjust one's lifestyle so that no tranquillising agents are needed.

DIET ADVICE Follow an optimum diet, avoiding all stimulants. Do not eat sugar or drink tea or coffee in the evening. Eat seeds, nuts and vegetables, which are high in calcium and magnesium.

SUPPLEMENTS 1 x Multivitamin; 1 x Zinc 10mg; 3 x Dolomite; 1 x B6 100mg; 1 x Vitamin C 1,000mg; 1 x B Complex 1 x Multimineral; 2 x L-Tryptophan 500mg (only if absolutely necessary)

Menstrual problems

Pre-menstrual problems as well as menopausal problems can be helped by optimum nutrition. Particularly important are vitamin B6, zinc, magnesium and essential fatty acids. While the need for these is greater in pre-menstrual tension before the period is due, it is wise to take the supplements throughout the month.

DIET ADVICE Follow an optimum diet. Ensure that your diet contains one tablespoon of cold-pressed vegetable oil.

SUPPLEMENTS 1 x Multivitamin; 2 x B6 100mg; 1 x Zinc 10mg; 1 x C 1,000mg; 1 x B Complex; 1 x Multimineral; 1 x GLA 150mg

Senility

Senility is primarily characterised by a loss of memory. While this may be caused in part by poor circulation, a decrease in the brain chemical acetylcholine is often found. Vitamin B5, as well as choline, are needed to produce acetylcholine so all these are recommended. Many other nutrients are also involved in maintaining optimum mental function. A hair mineral analysis can help determine if any toxic levels of metals are present, especially aluminium.

DIET ADVICE Follow an optimum diet, and be sure to drink plenty of water.

SUPPLEMENTS

1 x Multivitamin; 1 x B Complex; 1 x Vitamin B5 (Pantothenic acid) 500mg; 1 x Vitamin C 1,000mg; 1 x Multimineral
2 tablespoons of lecithin granules (on food)

Ulcers

Stomach ulcers occur in the stomach, and duodenal ulcers in the duodenum - the first section of the small intestine, which is not so well protected as the rest of the intestines against the acid secretions of the stomach. In prolonged stress the stomach can over-secrete acid so stress can be a cause. Also, diets that are too acid-forming are to be avoided.

This means eating less meat, fish and other high protein foods. Citrus fruit can also be irritating. Vitamin A is the primary nutrient needed to protect the lining of the duodenum. While vitamin C does help those with duodenal ulcers, not more than 500mg should be taken as it can cause irritation. If a burning sensation is experienced after taking vitamin C the dose is too high.

DIET ADVICE Follow the vitality diet, keeping mainly to alkaline forming foods.

SUPPLEMENTS 1 x Multi-vitamin; 2 x Vitamin A (as beta-carotene) 7,500iu; 1 x B Complex; 1 x Vitamin C 500mg; 1 x Multimineral

Vitamins for First Aid

Although on-going optimum nutrition will prepare you for accidents and emergencies, there are many situations in which optimum nutrition can provide immediate relief. All doses stated are for adults, and children's needs should be scaled down accordingly. **These doses are not intended for continuous use.**

Abscess A localised infection. Increase vitamin C intake to 1,000mg five times a day, and vitamin A (as beta carotene) in 7,500iu capsules to four capsules once a day for no more than one week. This will help strengthen your immune system. Vitamin B6 100mg twice a day helps to localise the infection and acts as a mild analgesic. Take a B Complex if you're on antibiotics.

Allergic Reaction Sudden allergies can occur because of something you have eaten or been exposed to. Take 500mg of vitamin B5 or 5,000mg of vitamin C and drink plenty of water. This will help you to return to normal. Dolomite powder (high in calcium and magnesium) also helps to restore balance. The same advice applies to hayfever.

Burns Burns need to be treated instantly. Don't put on plasters until the heat is out of the burn. To heal it take up to 20,000iu of vitamin A (as beta carotene) per day and 30mg of zinc for one week or less, depending on the burn. Vitamin E oil can be applied when the burn is not an open wound. Drink plenty of fluids.

Colds or Flu As soon as you feel the first signs of a cold or flu take two 1,000mg tablets of vitamin C every four hours. As soon as you no longer feel the symptoms, reduce to 1,000mg every four hours. Take 4,000mg daily for the next three days as a cold can be suppressed for this time. If you are able to saturate your bloodstream with vitamin C fast enough for long enough, most colds do not last. If you get abdominal discomfort you are taking too much. Eat little and certainly avoid sugar and alcohol.

Cuts and Bruises From a nutritional point of view, these are the same as burns. Scars from cuts heal up spectacularly well when you take 1,000iu of vitamin E and apply the oil to the injury site (but only when it is not an open wound).

Exhaustion Total exhaustion is a sign for you to take it easy. Take some days off and if you feel like just staying in bed, do so. Take 500mg of vitamin B5, 100mg of vitamin B3 (niacin) and 2,000mg of vitamin C three times a day for one day only. The B3 will cause a beneficial blushing effect. However, if you don't like it take niacinamide instead.

Hangover The symptoms of excess alcohol are half dehydration and half detoxification. So drink masses of liquids and take a B Complex and 2,000mg of vitamin C twice in the day. If you know you're going to be drinking a lot this is best done before your excesses.

Headaches These are often due to tension and maybe nature's way of slowing you down. Instead of taking an aspirin, or migraine drugs which constrict the blood vessels, try taking between 100 and 200mg of vitamin B3 niacin, which is a vaso-dilator. Start with the smaller dose. This will cause a 'blushing' sensation as well as increased heat and can often stop or reduce a migraine in the early stages.

Infections Increase vitamin C intake to 1,000mg five times a day and 30,000ius vitamin A (as beta carotene) for no more than one week. This will help strengthen your immune system. 100mg of vitamin B6 twice a day helps to localise the infection and acts as a mild analgesic. Take a B Complex if you're on antibiotics. Avoid sugar entirely and ensure that your diet is very healthy.

Leg Cramps Cramps are usually due to calcium/magnesium imbalances. Take 1,000mg of calcium and 500mg of magnesium. The condition is, very rarely, due to a lack of salt, after a long run in the heat, for example. Except in these circumstances, it is best to avoid added salt and keep fluid intake high.

Mouth Ulcers These are very often due either to an allergy or to lack of vitamin A or excess sugar from sweets. Take up to 20,000iu of vitamin A, as betacarotene a day. Wheat and grain allergies can also result in mouth ulcers.

Overdose Overdoses require immediate medical attention. However, an excess of cannabis, amphetamines, cocaine or LSD seriously depleted B vitamins so these must be restored immediately. For a 'bad trip' on LSD or psyllicybin mushrooms take 5,000mg of vitamin C immediately. Any smoking, whether of tobacco or anything else, destroys vitamin C. Take an extra 25mg for each cigarette you smoke, with a maximum daily intake of 4,000mg. Much more important is to stop the habit.

Shock Shock, such as in a car accident, causes a considerable release of adrenalin. Make sure you have the time and place to relax and ensure an intake of 3,000mg of vitamin C and two B Complex tablets over the day.

Stings Stings cause a histamine reaction that isolates the poison. Cooling the sting helps to reduce itchiness, as does taking 200mg of vitamin B6.

Sunburn Sunburn is best prevented by using a PABA sunscreen - the most effective sunscreen of all. But once you are burnt, follow the advice given for burns. If you have sensitive skin it is wise to ensure a daily intake of 100mg of PABA.

USEFUL ADDRESSES

THE BRITISH SOCIETY FOR NUTRITIONAL MEDICINE is concerned with nutrition as it relates to medical practice. Full membership is only open to medical practitioners. If your doctor is interested in optimum nutrition this is the best organisation for them to contact. *BSNM, PO Box 3AP, London W1A 3AP.*

THE INSTITUTE FOR OPTIMUM NUTRITION offers courses and personal consultations with qualified nutritionists, including Patrick Holford. On request ION will send you a free information pack. See page 159. *ION,5 Jerdan Place, London SW6 1BE Tel: 071 385 7984; Fax: 071 385 3249.*

THE NUTRITION CONSULTANTS ASSOCIATION is an association of qualified nutrition consultants trained at ION. They publish a directory of nutrition consultants throughout Great Britain which is available, either direct from them, or from ION for £1.50. *NCA c/o 5 Jerdan Place, London SW6 1BE.*

FORESIGHT provides information and personal advice on the importance of pre-conceptual care and nutrition. For more details send an SAE to *Foresight, The Old Vicarage, Church Lane, Witley, Godalming, Surrey GU8 5PN.*

HYPERACTIVE CHILDREN'S SUPPORT GROUP offer help and advice for the families of hyperactive children. Please send an SAE to *HACSG Mayfield House, Yapton Road, Barnham, Bognor Regis, West Sussex PO22 0BJ.*

DIRECTORY OF
SUPPLEMENT COMPANIES

The following supplement companies provide a wide range of supplements providing optimum levels of nutrients, as defined in this book. Most of these companies, and many health food shops, have staff on hand who can help you choose the best supplements to meet your needs.

Cantassium produce an extensive range of vitamin and mineral supplements, both through health food shops, and by mail order. Their best multivitamin is *Cantamega 2000*. Send for a free catalogue to: *Larkhall Natural Health, 225 Putney Bridge Road, London SW15 2PY (Tel: 081 874 1130)*.

Health+Plus produce an extensive range of vitamin and mineral supplements available by mail order. They have products suitable for specific dietary needs as well as their most popular multivitamin *The VV Pack*. Send for a free catalogue to: *Health+Plus, PO Box 86, Seaford, Sussex BN25 4ZW (Tel: 0323 492096)*.

Green Farm produce an extensive range of vitamin and mineral supplements available both through health food shops and by mail order. Their best multivitamin is the *Mega Multi*. Send for a free catalogue to: *Green Farm, Burwash Common, East Sussex TN19 7LX (Tel: 0435 882482)*. changed 081 874 1130

Nature's Best produce an extensive range of vitamin and mineral supplements available by mail order. Their best multivitamin is *Multi-Guard*. Write or phone for a free 76 page colour catalogue to: *Nature's Best Ltd, Freepost (Dept OH) PO Box 1, Tunbridge Wells TN2 3BR (Tel: 0892 534143)*.

Quest produce an extensive range of vitamin and mineral supplements available through health food shops. Their best multivitamin is *Super Once-A-Day*. In case of difficulty contact: *The Nutritionist, Quest Vitamins Ltd, Unit 1, Premier Trading Estate, Dartmouth Middleway, Birmingham B7 4AT (Tel: 021 359 0056) for your nearest stockist*.

Solgar produce an extensive range of vitamin and mineral supplements available through health food shops. Their best multivitamin is *VM2000*. In case of difficulty contact: *Solgar Vitamins, Solgar House, Chiltern Commerce Centre, Asheridge Road, Chesham, Bucks HP5 2PY (Tel: 0494 791691) for your nearest stockist*.

Winsor Health foods Winsor RG

INDEX